# Clean Start

Nancy Spiccia, CPA, CHC

Zabaglione Press

# DEDICATION

For all moms, who want to make the world a little safer & healthier place.
Never underestimate the influence you have. ❤

# CONTENTS

# ACKNOWLEDGMENTS

My Deepest Gratitude to:

Joseph, Susanna, Joe & Natalie
For your loving support throughout this process.

Jason Neubauer
For your beautiful cover design and photography.

Lindsey Smith and Joshua Rosenthal
For your encouragement, guidance & inspiration.

You are amazing. ❤

# 1 THE POLLUTED WORLD WE LIVE IN

## My Chemical Nightmare

It was one of the most surreal moments in my life as I stood backstage at the Dr. Oz Show in New York City, waiting for my cue to join Dr. Oz. I was there to discuss my own chemical nightmare before one of the largest viewing audiences in the world. Dr. Oz was warm and reassuring as he asked me about my personal experience with toxins and how they had wreaked havoc on my health. While all went well and they used my segment for their national commercial, I was struck by the gravity of what I had just shared. My body was filled with toxins, dangerous chemicals that are linked to cancer and other serious health problems. I knew these chemicals by name and they were residing inside of my body at alarming levels, despite years of medical intervention to attempt to remove them. As I thought about how my children had tested positive for many of these same toxins, I was hit by the sobering reality that I had passed on this chemical curse.

I couldn't help but wonder if my story was unique. I only became aware of these chemicals when my specific health problems prompted my doctors to conduct environmental toxicity testing. Maybe everyone was filled with many of these same chemicals to one degree or another. How many other mothers, like me, had also accumulated a high level of chemicals that they too would pass on to their children? Would they even want to know? Where do the chemicals come from and what health risks do they pose? Is there a way to remove them? Are some chemicals worse than others? My search for answers to these never-ending questions took me down a path of some startling discoveries about the world we live in.

## The Pollution in Newborn Babies

Once upon a time, scientists believed that the placentas of developing newborns shielded their tiny bodies from all of the environmental chemicals and pollutants in the world. Today we know from several shocking scientific studies that this is not the case. While our babies spend their first nine months of development in their mother's womb, they receive a constant supply of oxygen-rich blood that provides them with all of the building blocks for a healthy body. At the same time, they are receiving a steady flow of industrial chemicals and other serious pollutants through that same umbilical cord blood.

# A BENCHMARK INVESTIGATION OF INDUSTRIAL CHEMICALS, POLLUTANTS AND PESTICIDES IN UMBILICAL CORD BLOOD

*Environmental Working Group, July 14, 2005*

The Environmental Working Group (EWG) performed one of the first of several studies to test the umbilical cord blood of babies for chemicals, and the results gained significant attention from around the world. The study found an average of 287 different chemicals from numerous pesticides, consumer product ingredients, waste from burning coal, gasoline, and garbage. They included chemicals found in Teflon™, flame retardants, mercury, lead, BPA, phthalates, DDT, and benzene, which are all known to be extremely hazardous to human health.

Of the 287 chemicals detected:
- 180 were linked to cancer in humans or animals
- 217 are considered toxic to the brain and nervous system
- 208 have been linked to birth defects or abnormal development

According to a senior scientist for this study, "We know the developing fetus is one of the most vulnerable populations, if not the most vulnerable, to environmental exposure. Their organ systems aren't mature and their detox methods are not in place, so cord blood gives us a good picture of exposure during this most vulnerable time of life."

## Our Environment is Changing

No mother would intentionally expose her baby to toxic chemicals, yet in today's world, it's become impossible to completely avoid the chemicals that have been introduced into our environment. Most of these chemicals were unheard of 150 years ago.

The widespread development and use of chemicals in the late twentieth century has changed our planet forever, and today there doesn't appear to be one place left on earth that is not contaminated. We live in a man-made polluted environment that is affecting us all on a daily basis, most of which is invisible to the human eye, making it easier for us to believe that we are not being affected.

Many people believe that the government regulates the chemicals in our food and consumer products to protect us from these toxins. This couldn't be further from the truth when you consider that there are now over 80,000 chemicals registered with the EPA in the United States and less than 500 have been tested for toxicity.

What's really scary is that we're seeing a cumulative effect as chemicals are silently passed on from one generation to another. These chemicals are affecting our gene expression, or our "epigenetics," a field that is gaining tremendous attention in the scientific community today.

## How Do These Chemicals Get Into Our Bodies?

After our initial exposure to chemicals through umbilical cord blood in utero, our exposure to toxins continues until the day we die. The main way chemicals enter our body is through what we eat and drink, but we also absorb them through our skin and through the air we breath.

We are eating chemicals as pesticides, additives, and preservatives. Our food packaging materials, such as plastics, are leaching chemicals into our food. We're drinking them in our tap water and absorbing them into our skin from our cosmetics, shampoos, and the lotions we put on our bodies every day. We absorb the fire retardants in our mattresses, and other chemicals from the clothing we wear. We breathe in gases that come from our furniture, shower curtains, carpets, treated wood, and swimming pools. We even inhale them in the air when we fill our cars with gas, breathe in exhaust fumes, perfumes, air fresheners, and everyday cleaning products. There are really very few places left to hide.

## So What Chemicals Are We Talking About?

There are basically two main groups of chemicals that appear to be causing so many of the health problems we're facing today: toxic heavy metals and synthetic chemicals.

Toxic heavy metals are part of our natural environment and they have been around a long time. The problem is that we've seen an explosive increase in these chemicals as a result of increased manufacturing and other human activities, and our natural detoxification mechanisms are just not able to handle these high levels of exposure. Heavy metals include chemicals such as mercury, lead, cadmium, chromium, arsenic, and manganese. Common sources are from industrial wastes, vehicle emissions, fertilizers, lead-acid batteries, treated wood, and paints.

# Lead

The most prevalent heavy metal contaminant is lead, which was used extensively in gasoline until the 1970s. Today lead levels remain high in the aquatic environments of industrialized nations. And even though lead was banned from use in the United States in 1996, concentrations still remain high in the soil near roads that were built before this time.

Lead exposure is also imported from foreign countries like China, including toys that our children play with and put into their mouths. We're hearing about recalls quite often, but only after tragedy has struck.

According to the EPA, "lead poses a significant health risk to young children, especially infants and fetuses, where the danger is very severe. This is because growing children absorb lead more rapidly and are negatively impacted by a level of lead exposure that would have little effect on an adult. A child's mental and physical development can be irreversibly impaired by over-exposure to lead." The EPA estimates that drinking water can account for 20% or more of a person's lead exposure. Infants who consume formula mixed with drinking water can be exposed to lead at much higher levels (from 40% to 60%) when the formula is their primary source of nourishment. (40)

# Mercury

Warnings about mercury in seafood have gained significant attention in recent years due to the serious health risks associated with this toxic heavy metal. The two largest sources for mercury exposure are through air and water. A recent study published in the Journal of Environmental Monitoring (3) found that mercury in the atmosphere is one of the most ignored sources of air pollution, and it reaches particularly dangerous levels in urban areas. Many experts feel that the EPA has been lax in enforcing mercury-pollution standards, which has led to a serious increase in the problem.

Because mercury is a neurotoxin, it can cause serious harm to the developing brains of babies in utero as well as infants and children. It's also been linked to memory loss, infertility, and an increase in blood pressure in adults. According to the EPA, exposures to mercury can affect the human nervous system and harm the brain, heart, kidneys, lungs, and immune system. The EPA also stated, "Some communities eat significantly higher quantities of fish than the general population, and thus may be exposed to much greater mercury contamination than the general population.

In addition, in past outbreaks of methylmercury poisoning, mothers with no symptoms of nervous system damage gave birth to infants with severe disabilities; as a result, it became clear that the nervous system of a developing fetus may be more vulnerable to methylmercury exposures than the adult nervous system. Mothers who are exposed to methylmercury and breast-feed may also expose their infant children through their milk." (40)

Some major sources of mercury in the environment include:
- Coal-burning power plants
- Chlor-alkali plants
- Gold mining
- Trash incinerators
- Cement kilns

Common sources of mercury in consumer products include:
- **Fish and Seafood** (and animals that eat seafood)
- **Dental amalgam fillings** – This material is made of 40-50% mercury, 25% silver and 25-35% a mixture of copper, zinc and tin. Use is declining due to controversy regarding safety as well the availability of effective alternative materials that appear more natural. Learn more from the IAOMT (International Academy of Oral Medicine and Toxicology), a nonprofit organization of dentists who are concerned about the safe use and removal of amalgam fillings @ http://iaomt.org.
- **Fever thermometers** - In 2008, thirteen states passed laws limiting their manufacture, sale or distribution: California, Connecticut, Illinois, Indiana, Maine, Maryland, Massachusetts, Michigan, Minnesota, New Hampshire, Rhode Island, Oregon, Washington.
- **Antiques** – Some clocks, barometers, and mirrors contain elemental mercury
- **Batteries** - Most batteries made in the U.S. today do not contain added mercury, with two exceptions: mercuric oxide batteries & button cell batteries.
- **CFLs and Other Fluorescent Light Bulbs**- Save $ and electricity, but these release mercury when broken or improperly disposed of. Many are unaware of the need to immediately ventilate a room for a broken bulb and follow safety instructions on the product label.
- **Necklaces and Other Jewelry** - Some necklaces imported from Mexico contain a glass pendant that contains mercury. These come in various shapes such as hearts, bottles, balls, saber teeth, and chili peppers. If broken, they release dangerous metallic mercury.

- **Paint**- Previously used extensively in interior & exterior paint and fungicides to prevent bacteria growth. Discontinued in the U.S. in 1991 for interior/exterior paints. Be careful with remodeling of older homes and buildings.
- **Skin-Lightening Creams** – Numerous cases of mercury poisoning have been investigated by the FDA due to the use of creams used for lightening the skin, fading freckles and age spots, and treating acne. Creams imported from Mexico and the Dominican Republic may contain thousands of times the level of mercury allowed by the U.S. FDA.
- **Switches and Relays**
- **Thermostats** – While unlikely to break or leak mercury while in use, they must be properly disposed of when being replaced by taking them to a state or local household hazardous waste collection center for recycling.
- **Thimerosal in Vaccines** – This mercury-containing preservative has been removed from many vaccines due to considerable controversy over safety. The flu (influenza) vaccine still contains thimerosal. Travelers to high-risk countries requiring vaccines can sometimes find thimerosal-free options.

According to the EPA, the most dangerous exposures of mercury occur when we breathe mercury vapor. It's important to ventilate a room immediately when mercury is present (i.e. broken CFL light bulb).

## Synthetic Chemicals

Synthetic chemicals, manufactured in laboratories in massive quantities have widespread use today with the potential for levels of unprecedented toxicity. These chemicals are found in things we use every day, including many of our drugs, cleaning products, shampoos, lotions, nail polish, pesticides in our food, dry cleaning solvents, rubber, food preservatives, and food coloring. Unlike heavy metals, we have no way of dealing with many of these chemicals and unfortunately, they have nowhere to go but into our bodies where they accumulate over our lifetime. Our best defense is to avoid them as much as possible.

Let's stop and take a deep breath. While it's important to understand what chemicals we're dealing with, we're going to look at some of the most common sources for exposure and what we can do minimize our risk. Our simple choices can really make a difference!

## So What Chemicals Were Found in Newborn Babies?

Let's take a look at the specific chemicals identified in the Newborn Study of Umbilical Cord Blood, (1) so we'll have a better idea of some common exposures that our children may be dealing with:

**Chemicals Identified:**

- **Mercury (Hg) – tested for 1, found 1**
  Pollutant from coal-fired power plants, mercury-containing products, and certain industrial processes. Accumulates in seafood.
  Harms brain development and function.

- **Polyaromatic hydrocarbons (PAHs) - tested for 18, found 9**
  Pollutants from burning gasoline and garbage. Accumulates in food chain.
  Linked to cancer.

- **Polybrominated dibenzodioxins & furans (PBDD/F) tested for 12, found 7** Contaminants in brominated flame retardants. Pollutants and byproducts from plastic production and incineration. Accumulate in food chain.
  Toxic to developing endocrine (hormone) system.

- **Perfluorinated chemicals (PFCs) - tested for 12, found 9**
  Active ingredients or breakdown products of Teflon™, Scotchgard™, fabric and carpet protectors, food wrap coatings, and global contaminants. Accumulate in the environment and the food chain.
  Linked to cancer, birth defects, and more.

- **Polychlorinated dibenzodioxins & furans (PBCD/F) tested for 17, found 11**
  Pollutants, by-products of PVC production, industrial bleaching, and incineration. Persist for decades in the environment.
  Cause cancer in humans.
  Very toxic to developing endocrine (hormone) system.

- **Organochlorine pesticides (OCs) - tested for 28, found 21**
  DDT, chlordane, and other pesticides. Largely banned in the U.S. yet persist for decades in the environment. Accumulate up the food chain, to man.
  Cause cancer and numerous reproductive issues.

- **Polybrominated diphenyl ethers (PBDEs) - tested for 46, found 32**
  Flame retardant in furniture foam, computers, and televisions. Accumulates in the food chain and human tissues.
  Adversely affects brain development and the thyroid.

- **Polychlorinated Naphthalenes (PCNs) - tested for 70, found 50**
  Wood preservatives, varnishes, machine lubricating oils, waste incineration. Common PCB contaminant. Contaminate the food chain.
  Cause liver and kidney damage.

- **Polychlorinated biphenyls (PCBs) - tested for 209, found 147**
  Industrial insulators and lubricants. Banned in the U.S. in 1976 yet persist for decades in the environment. Accumulate up the food chain, to man.
  Cause cancer and nervous system problems.

## Consider the State of Our Health Today

Our body's immune system is a complicated network of cells, tissues, and organs that work around the clock to keep us healthy and help to fight off disease and infection. We know that many factors contribute to having a healthy immune system, including the amount of stress our bodies are up against. Factors such as chemical exposure, radiation, and exposure to certain diseases can cause the immune system to deteriorate. The food we eat is one of the most basic building blocks for creating a healthy immune system that will enable our bodies to properly detoxify and rebuild healthy cells.

Unfortunately, our super-busy lifestyles drive us to make compromises for convenience with regard to what we eat and what we feed our families. These foods often contain high levels of sugar, fat and artificial ingredients that are creating serious health problems.

Fast food sales have increased nearly 2000% over the past 30 years and have been linked to acute inflammation, putting our families at increased risk for heart disease, type 2 diabetes, arthritis, certain cancers, and neurological dysfunction. Asthma has skyrocketed since 1980, reaching epidemic levels. Type 2 Diabetes can no longer be called "Adult-Onset" diabetes because it's now a common problem found in children as well as adults.

Marketing has lead to meals that cater specifically to children by luring them with toys and prizes connected to nutritionally deficient food. It's become a norm for many parents to feed their children a different meal (often less nutritious) than they're eating. We're raising a nation of children with emotional and psychological connections to junk food that is severely lacking in nutrition.

The standard American diet (S.A.D.) has resulted in a nation filled with overfed yet undernourished people. How do we expect our children to thrive in a world inundated with so many chemicals, many of which they are ingesting as part of their everyday diet?

## The Obesity Epidemic

According to the American Heart Association 2011 Statistical Sourcebook:

- About 1 in 3 children and teens in the U.S. is overweight or obese.
- Overweight kids have a 70–80 percent chance of staying overweight their entire lives.
- Obese and overweight adults now outnumber those at a healthy weight; nearly 7 in 10 U.S. adults are overweight or obese.

## Health Effects of Childhood Obesity

According to the Centers for Disease Control (cdc.org), childhood obesity has both immediate and long-term effects on health and wellbeing.

Immediate health effects:

- Obese youth are more likely to have risk factors for cardiovascular disease, such as high cholesterol or high blood pressure. In a population-based sample of 5- to 17-year-olds, 70% of obese youth had at least one risk factor for cardiovascular disease.[4]

- Obese adolescents are more likely to have pre-diabetes, a condition in which blood glucose levels indicate a high risk for development of diabetes.[5,6]

- Children and adolescents who are obese are at greater risk for bone and joint problems, sleep apnea, and social and psychological problems such as stigmatization and poor self-esteem. [7,8,9]

Long-term health effects:

- Children and adolescents who are obese are likely to be obese as adults and are therefore, more at risk for adult health problems such as heart disease, type 2 diabetes, stroke, several types of cancer, and osteo-arthritis.(6) One study showed that children who became obese as early as age 2 were more likely to be obese as adults.(10)

- Overweight and obesity are associated with increased risk for many types of cancer, including cancer of the breast, colon, endometrium, esophagus, kidney, pancreas, gall bladder, thyroid, ovary, cervix, and prostate, as well as multiple myeloma and Hodgkin's lymphoma. (11)

## Making Changes For Our Children's Sake

The American Academy of Pediatrics issued a statement recently that suggests that unless current trends reverse, **one in three children born today can expect a shorter life than their parents**!

Our children are facing some very serious health challenges today. As parents, we have a responsibility to our children and to future generations to do all that we can to establish healthy habits and to limit their exposure to toxic chemicals. What a gift we can give our children when from the very start of their lives, we provide them every advantage to thrive. ♥

---

*"Whenever I held my newborn baby in my arms, I used to think that what I said and did to him could have an influence not only on him but on all whom he met, not only for a day or a month or a year, but for all eternity – a very challenging and exciting thought for a mother."* - Rose Kennedy

---

# 2 SMALL CHANGES – BIG IMPACT

*"You'll never change your life until you change something you do daily. The secret of your success is found in your daily routine." --John Maxwell*

## Genes Are Not Destiny

While our world is radically changing and the challenges we face today may seem overwhelming, we actually have a lot more control than we may think. Scientists have recently shown that we are not merely victims of the genes we've inherited from our parents. Instead, we now know that our lifestyle and environment actually have a profound impact on how our genes are expressed, our "epigenetics" (meaning "above genetics"). In other words, while our genes may set the stage for our susceptibility to developing a particular disease, whether we actually get that disease is largely determined by factors associated with our lifestyle and environment, from the things we eat, to the pollution we're exposed to, to the impact of stress in our lives. Our lifestyle choices can influence our gene activity without changing our actual DNA. They influence how our genetic code is expressed: whether each gene is turned on or off, how each gene is strengthened or weakened, which in turn affects everything in our bodies. One way to look at it is that our genes load the gun, while our environment and lifestyle pull the trigger.

Epigenetics considers what happens to our genes over the course of our lifetime and whether those changes can be passed down to our children, or even our grandchildren through "epigenetic marks" on our DNA. There is evidence that this may in fact be the case, and if so, parents may find themselves responsible for passing on the effects of their poor lifestyle habits to future generations.

## The Statistics Are Screaming Prevention!

While the levels of health problems we're facing today have reached epidemic proportions, there is some good news! The leading causes of death are largely **preventable** through healthy lifestyle choices!

Heart Disease:

The American Heart Association has stated that 80% of heart disease is preventable with proper nutrition and healthy lifestyle choices (12).

Type 2 Diabetes:

If type 2 diabetes was an infectious disease, public health officials would say we're in the midst of an epidemic. Once called "adult-onset diabetes," the name change reflects the alarming number of teenagers and children who now have it. According to the Harvard School of Public Health, "about 9 cases in 10 could be avoided by taking several simple steps: keeping weight under control, exercising more, eating a healthy diet, and not smoking." (13)

Cancer:

The American Association for Cancer Research (AACR) just released its annual Cancer Progress report (14) stating, "Cancer cases are also expected to grow by 33% over the next 20 years, topping off at 2.4 million. However, the good news is that more than half of all diagnosed cases can be attributed to preventable causes." They go on to say, once again, that lifestyle choices matter. In fact, they are a matter of life and death.

## Think Cumulative

Overhauling your lifestyle all at once is probably unrealistic, especially when unhealthy habits are well established. It's important to remember that even the small changes we make daily lives can add up—they can have a cumulative affect with the potential to make a huge impact over time. If you find yourself getting overwhelmed, just cut yourself some slack and remember, we're all on a journey to better health. Be gentle with yourself and others as you move toward your goals and always let love be your motivation. ❤

# 3 CLEAN EATING

"Clean eating" or "eating clean" is a term you've probably heard a lot these days. It's become a major movement that is fueled by people who want to feel good about what they're putting in their bodies. It's about being mindful of where your food has come from and choosing foods in their most natural form. Someone who eats clean prefers real or whole foods over processed foods. They are conscious of the toxins associated with their food choices.

We'll spend a little time focusing on some of the major areas of clean eating as well as how to identify the cleanest sources of different types of food. These will include produce, meat and poultry, fish, and dairy products. We'll also talk about a hot topic that has provoked considerable controversy: genetically modified organisms, or GMOs.

## Eat Real Food

Eating clean begins with making healthy choices. One of the most important things we can do for our health is to eat more real food, including a rainbow of wholesome fresh fruits and vegetables, preferably from local sources and in season, whole grains and only meat, poultry and fish from clean, sustainable sources.

Real food is about enjoying delicious, wholesome, healthy food in its most natural state. It can be minimally processed, such as chopping up fruit, and it's still considered wholesome. What we want to avoid are foods that are processed in a way that reduce their nutritional value, such as taking rice in it's natural form (brown) and putting it through a mechanical process to remove the fiber (now white). Processing depletes a food of the nutrients it was intended to provide. Often these foods are "enriched" with synthetic nutrients that do not promote health in the same way as those provided in their natural state.

The most highly processed foods often contain chemical preservatives, artificial colorings, food additives, or flavorings. These are designed to have a longer shelf life than real food, but they come with a high price tag with regard to our health. The more ingredients you see on the label, the more processed it usually is. Processed foods are often high in sugar, low in fiber, high in sodium, and contain unhealthy fats that will wreak havoc on your family's health. When we feed our children processed food, we increase their body burden by allowing more toxic chemicals to enter their body. In contrast, the cleaner our food choices, the more we equip our children with nutrients that promote health and encourage natural detoxification.

The key to eating healthy food is knowing where your food came from and what's in it, and the easiest way to do that is to cook at home as often as possible. It's not only healthier since you know exactly what you're getting, but you'll get far more quality for the money you spend.

## Become a Label Reader

By the time my third child was in preschool, I had become much more aware of what I was feeding my family. I became an avid label reader and taught my daughter what to look for on a label. I'll never forget the day she picked up a box in our grocery cart and told me not to buy it because it had MSG (monosodium glutamate--a flavor enhancer that many experts believe is one of the worst food additives on the market). A woman nearby couldn't believe what she had heard and commented on what a great job I was doing as a mom. That was a proud day.

Sometimes we're so busy that we forget that our children are like sponges soaking in all that we share with them. They have a tremendous capacity and desire to learn, so let's take advantage of the precious time we have with them, while they are listening.

## Sugar is Toxic

Americans are eating more sugar than ever and the trend doesn't appear to be stopping anytime soon. This dramatic rise in sugar consumption is driven by the industrialization and commercialization of our food, primarily through large manufacturers who are more interested in profit than they are in public health. Unfortunately, the over-consumption of sugar is behind many of today's serious health issues.

According to Mark Hyman, MD, author of *The Blood Sugar Solution*, "The facts are in, the science is beyond question. Sugar in all its forms is the root cause of our obesity epidemic and most of the chronic disease sucking the life out of our citizens and our economy — and, increasingly, the rest of the world. You name it, it's caused by sugar: heart disease, cancer, dementia, type 2 diabetes, depression, and even acne, infertility and impotence."

Dr. Hyman goes on to say, "The average American consumes about 152 pounds of sugar a year. That's roughly 22 teaspoons every day for every person in America. And our kids consume about 34 teaspoons every day — that's more than two 20-ounce sodas — making nearly 1 in 4 teenagers pre-diabetic or diabetic."

Not only does sugar alter gene expression and negatively affect several biochemical pathways – according to a 2007 study (2), it was found to be more addictive than cocaine!

## Sneaky Hidden Sugar in Food

Do you have any idea how much sugar your family is eating? To be able to answer that question, you'll have to know the sources of sugar in your family's diet. Many people do not realize their level of sugar intake because it's hidden in so many foods.

While we expect to find sugar in cookies and ice cream, who would have thought we'd find quite a bit of it in ketchup, bread or spaghetti sauce? Some of the less obvious places to find sugar are in reduced-fat products such as peanut butter, since sugar is added to compensate for the lack of flavor resulting from fat removal. If we want to set our kids up for a healthier future, then it's very important that we consider how much sugar they are getting and make some changes. The more we move towards reducing sugar, the better off our families will be long-term.

## Create A Sugar Reduction Strategy

If sugar was found to be more addictive than cocaine, then it's reasonable to assume that it may not be easy to stop eating it cold turkey. It's reasonable to assume that if your children eat a lot of sugar, they will put up a fight if you cut all sources off quickly. It may be better to make a strategic plan for reducing sugar over time and make it positive. Have fun with your kids by making "spritzers" or "soda" using sparkling water and a shot of unsweetened fruit juice. Try cutting back on sugar in recipes. Most recipes will still taste great when you cut the sugar by a third or even in half. You can reduce your family's sugar intake by taking small steps every day. You'll likely notice changes in mood and behavior as you move towards less sugar. Less sugar is good in so many ways.

One of the most important ways to identify hidden sugar in products is to read the label. Sugar goes by many names and companies have learned how to hide it by using several sources in one product. When you read a label, the most abundant ingredients are listed first. If you see the real food listed near the end and sugar is at the beginning, beware.

If a food has high fructose corn syrup, just put it back. High fructose corn syrup is always found in very poor-quality foods that are nutritionally deficient, often along with bad fats, excess salt, chemicals, and even mercury. It has devastating effects on metabolism.

Get to know the many alternative names for sugar. If something ends in "ose" or "ols", they generally are forms of sugar. Here are some forms of sugar you'll see on a label:

- agave
- brown sugar
- cane juice
- cane syrup
- corn sweetener
- crystalline fructose
- dextrose
- evaporated cane juice
- fructose
- fruit juice concentrates
- glucose
- honey
- high-fructose corn syrup
- invert sugar
- lactose
- maltose
- malt syrup
- molasses
- raw sugar
- sucrose
- syrup

Even more sneaky are the "ols" which are basically sugar alcohols. You can find these in a lot of chewing gum and breath mints. They include:

- sorbitol
- xylitol
- mannitol
- maltitol

While many believe that artificial sweeteners are a better choice than sugar, you may want to think twice about giving these controversial chemicals to your children. Small amount of sweeteners such as honey or real maple syrup may be a better choice, and stevia is considered by most experts to be a safe, natural alternative.

Experts previously recommended that no more than 10% of our calories should come from sugar, but the World Health Organization recently said we should slash that number even further to no more than 5% of our daily calories coming from sugar.

| Tips to Reduce Sugar Intake | |
|---|---|
| **Instead Of** | **Switch To** |
| Soft Drinks & Fruit Juice | Sparkling Water sweetened with small amount of unsweetened fruit juice; water with orange, lemon or lime slices. Wean from fruit juice by cutting with water & only use un-sweetened. Make it fun with "soda" or "spritzers" in special glasses. |
| Sweetened Frozen or Canned Fruit | Fresh or unsweetened frozen fruit |
| Yogurt (sweetened) | Organic Greek yogurt, sweeten plain with fruit. Transition by mixing ½ & ½ until phase out |
| Flavored Instant Oatmeal | Make your own oatmeal (fast, cheaper, tastes better, healthier). Sweeten with fruit, cinnamon, nuts, small amount honey/maple syrup. |
| Vanilla Almond Milk (sweetened) | Unsweetened vanilla |
| Peanut Butter | Natural Peanut Butter or Almond Butter, unsweetened |
| Jelly or Jam | All-fruit jams or warm up frozen berries |
| Spaghetti Sauce (jar) | Homemade Sauce- freeze extra for another use, better & save $ |
| Sweetened Cereal | Unsweetened cereal w/fruit |
| Cookies, chips, cakes, energy bars | Homemade trail mix, apple slices with peanut butter, carrots & humus, homemade protein bars. Be creative! |
| Sweetened Applesauce | Organic Unsweetened Apple Sauce (Apples are part of the "Dirty Dozen Plus"- see page 20). |

# Beware of Food Additives

Although processed and packaged foods may be convenient, they often contain thousands of food additives and preservatives to control shelf life, add color, flavor, nutrition, texture, aroma, and even to create addiction. Many of these should be avoided, especially since they can have a greater impact on children compared to adults and have been linked to things like ADHD and obesity. Because there are so many, I've listed some that are of particular concern. According to pediatrician Dr. Alan Greene, (26) we should be particularly attentive to these top five risky additives:

1. Artificial Colors – anything that begins with FD&C  (e.g. FD&C Blue No. 1)
2. Chemical Preservatives – Butylated Hydroxyanisole (BHA), Sodium Nitrate, Sodium Benzoate
3. Artificial Sweeteners – Aspartame, Acesulfame-K, Saccharin
4. Added Sugar – High Fructose Corn Syrup (HFCS), Corn Syrup, Dextrose, etc.
5. Added Salt – Look at the sodium content and choose foods with the lowest amounts.

Additionally, according to the Center for Science in the Public Interest, the following additives have been associated with negative health impacts:

- Propyl Gallate
- Sulfites (Sulfur Dioxide, Sodium Sulfite, Sodium/Potassium Bisulfite, Sodium and Potassium Metabisulfite)
- Potassium Bromate
- Monosodium Glutamate (MSG)
- Hydrogenated Vegetable Oil
- Partially Hydrogenated Vegetable Oil
- Potassium Bromate
- Olestra (Olean)
- Heptylparaben
- Sodium Nitrite

# Bug Spray for Dinner Anyone?

By the end of the nineteenth century, scientists had created synthetic chemicals that they discovered had the potential to impact human life. These chemicals were used as a part of chemical warfare until after the

Second World War when they needed to find alternative uses for the massive amounts of chemicals that had been produced. This led to a newly discovered use as pesticides in the farming community, which at the time, made economic sense to farmers who wanted to reduce their crop damage. This was the birth of conventional farming.

Because of this fundamental change in farming practices, we now have to face the fact that our food today is sprayed with many different toxic chemicals that include insecticides, fungicides, herbicides (weed killers), antibacterials, and rodenticides (kills rodents). These chemicals are undetectable to humans.

Many common fruits and vegetables are not only sprayed with multiple pesticides while they are growing, but they are sprayed again after harvesting to preserve them for shipping and storage, and even again before being packaged.

A study at California University in Davis (27) found that pre-school children who are exposed to pesticides are particularly at risk for developing cancer later in life. The study of 364 children (207 of whom were under the age of 5), found that safety levels were exceeded for arsenic, dioxins, dieldrin, and DDE and more than 95 per cent of pre-school children exceeded non-cancer risk levels for acrylamide - a cooking byproduct that is found in processed foods like potato chips and tortilla chips. According to the study, non-cancer risks include the death of cells.

The study also showed that pesticide levels were particularly high in peaches, apples, grapes, lettuce, strawberries, spinach, dairy, pears, peppers, green beans, celery, and broccoli.

The study leader, Dr. Rainbow Vogt stated, "We focused on children because early exposure can have long-term effects on disease outcomes. Currently the US Environmental Protection Agency only measures risk based on exposures of individual contaminants. We wanted to understand the cumulative risk from dietary contaminants. The results of this study demonstrate a need to prevent exposure to multiple toxins in young children to lower their cancer risk."

Recent government testing of produce showed that 2/3 of produce samples had pesticide residues. (28) No one wants to feed their family bug and weed killers, so let's consider how to make safer choices.

# When Organic Really Matters

The Environmental Working Group (EWG), a non-profit organization made up of scientists, researchers and policymakers, publishes an annual "Shopper's Guide to Pesticides in Produce." The guide includes two lists: "The Dirty Dozen Plus" and "The Clean 15," both of which are designed to help consumers decide when it's important to buy organic and when it's unnecessary.

## Does Washing Them Help?

These lists were compiled from data reported by the United States Department of Agriculture (USDA) after testing the amount of pesticide residue found on non-organic fruits and vegetables washed with high-powered water systems. While experts still recommend washing conventionally grown produce to remove residues, it's important to note that even after washing the fruits and vegetables on "The Dirty Dozen Plus" list, they still tested positive for at least 47 different chemicals, and some for as many as 67. According to Richard Wiles, senior vice president of policy for the EWG, "You should do what you can do, but the idea you are going to wash pesticides off is a fantasy."

According to the EWG, you can reduce the amount of toxins consumed on a daily basis by as much as 80% by eating certain types of organic produce. WOW! Needless to say, when choosing produce that is on "The Dirty Dozen Plus" list, organic is the way to go.

**2014 Dirty Dozen Plus**
1. Apples
2. Strawberries
3. Grapes
4. Celery
5. Peaches
6. Spinach
7. Sweet Bell Peppers
8. Nectarines (Imported)
9. Cucumbers
10. Cherry Tomatoes
11. Snap Peas (Imported)
12. Potatoes + Hot Peppers + Kale/Collard Greens

Nonorganic apples topped The EWG's Shopper's Guide to Pesticides in Produce for the fourth year in a row. Hot peppers, kale, and collard greens are frequently contaminated with insecticides that are toxic to human health, prompting their "Dirty Dozen Plus" status.

It's not all bad news! When deciding how to spend your money, keep in mind that the "Clean 15" have substantially lower pesticide levels than the "Dirty Dozen."

### 2014 Clean 15
These produce picks contained the lowest pesticide levels.
1. Avocados
2. Sweet Corn
3. Pineapples
4. Cabbage
5. Sweet Peas (Frozen)
6. Onions
7. Asparagus
8. Mangoes
9. Papayas
10. Kiwi
11. Eggplant
12. Grapefruit
13. Cantaloupe
14. Cauliflower
15. Sweet Potatoes

Check out the full list from on the Environmental Working Group's website: www.foodnews.org. You'll find some very handy tools to help you in the grocery store!

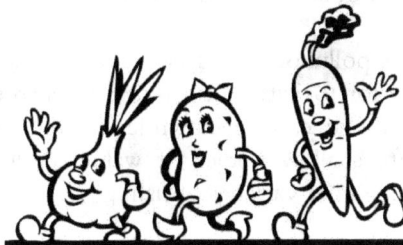

# Fish: A Mixed Bag

Fish and shellfish have long been considered healthy sources of protein throughout the world because of their high protein concentration and beneficial omega-3 fatty acids, EPA (eicosapentaenoic acid) and DHA (docosahexaenoic acid). Omega 3's have significant anti-inflammatory benefits that play a critical role in brain development, cognitive function and may play a significant role in preventing diabetes, heart disease, and Alzheimer's.

Despite the health benefits, there is growing concern about the safety of consuming fish since nearly all fish and shellfish contain serious pollutants found in our oceans, lakes, and streams due to environmental pollution. This pollution has come from many sources including everything from oil spills, industrial wastes, and even radioactive materials. It's still unclear how major disasters, such as the 2011 Japanese nuclear disaster in Fukushima resulting in radioactive water contamination, will affect marine life and humans.

Many people are shifting towards eating more vegetable sources to get their Omega 3's, although they do not provide the same level of quality as those found in fish. If you want to be sure that you're getting enough Omega 3's through vegetable sources (i.e. chia, walnuts, hemp, etc.), then you may want to ask your doctor for a simple blood test to measure your Omega 3 index level in red blood cell membranes.

## Most Fish Are Polluted With Traces Of Methylmercury

Mercury accumulates in fish when they swim in polluted water that is filtered through their gills. Mercury moves up the food chain and accumulates when larger fish eat smaller fish and add whatever levels of mercury are in the smaller fish to their own mercury level. The longer a fish lives, the greater the toxic accumulation, as is the case in humans who can accumulate the mercury of all the fish eaten during our lifetime.

The level of water pollution varies depending on where a fish swims, which is a key factor for toxicity. Fish found in deep cold water off the shores of Alaska, for instance, have shown less mercury accumulation than fish in warmer, more shallow bodies of water, an important factor to consider when choosing safer varieties of fish.

For years the Food and Drug Administration (FDA) and the Environmental Protection Agency (EPA) have issued warnings to pregnant and nursing women regarding their fish intake, however, in light of the current overwhelming science regarding the major health benefits of Omega 3's, they have recently (2014) issued an updated draft with recommendations that include **eating more fish that is lower in mercury** (at least 8oz and up to 12oz a week) in order to gain the developmental health benefits. (29)

Many experts are questioning this logic since there is conclusive evidence that there is enough mercury in most fish to harm the developing nervous system of an unborn baby or young child. If something can damage a fetus and cause learning abnormalities in children, then we have to ask ourselves if the benefits of eating it are worth the risks.

We may want to consider alternative sources of Omega 3s, including pharmaceutical grade purified fish oil supplements and vegetarian sources (i.e. flax seeds, chia seeds, walnuts, etc.). If you're pregnant, you'll have to decide your own personal level of comfort with regard to this issue.

The updated draft from the FDA and EPA warns pregnant and breastfeeding women to specifically avoid 4 types of fish that are associated with **high mercury levels:**

- Tilefish from the Gulf of Mexico
- Shark
- Swordfish
- King Mackerel
- Limit White (Albacore) Tuna to 6 ounces a week

Fish considered **lower in mercury** per their report include:

- Shrimp
- Pollock
- Salmon
- Canned light tuna
- Tilapia
- Catfish
- Cod

The update also recommended following fish advisories from local authorities when eating fish caught from local streams, rivers, and lakes. When that advice isn't available, they recommend limiting your total intake of such fish to 6 ounces a week for adults and 1-3 ounces for children.

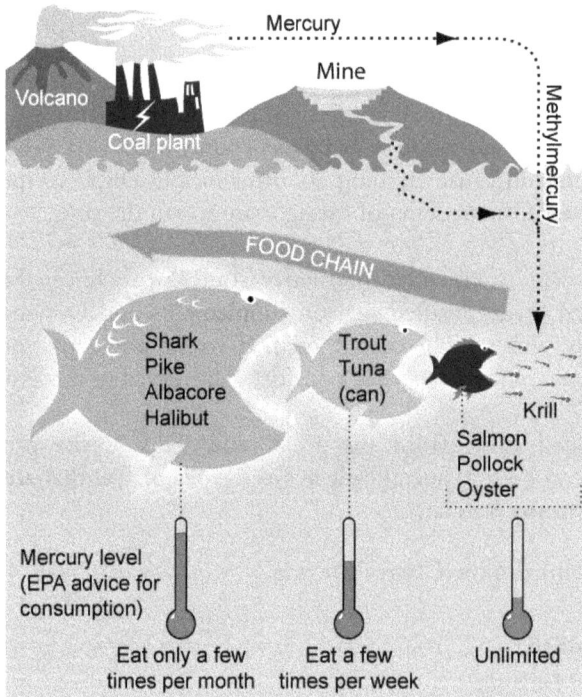

Mercury

Mine

Volcano

Coal plant

Methylmercury

FOOD CHAIN

Shark
Pike
Albacore
Halibut

Trout
Tuna
(can)

Krill

Salmon
Pollock
Oyster

Mercury level
(EPA advice for
consumption)

Eat only a few
times per month

Eat a few
times per week

Unlimited

Source: http://www.groundtruthtrekking.org/Graphics/MercuryFoodChain.html

## How Much Mercury Is In Seafood?

The following chart reflects the levels of mercury and Omega 3 fatty acids in specific varieties of fish, adapted from *The 2010 Dietary Guidelines for Americans*, (published by the USDA, 7th edition released since 1980 and will remain the current edition until the 2015 Dietary Guidelines for Americans is released). (30)

| Common Varieties Fish | Milligrams of Omega-3 Fatty Acids (EPA) and (DHA) Per 4 Ounces of Cooked Fish | Micrograms of Mercury Per 4 oz of Cooked Fish |
|---|---|---|
| Salmon: Atlantic, Chinook, Coho | 1200-2400 | 2 |
| Anchovies, Herring, Shad | 2300-2400 | 5-10 |
| Mackerel: Atlantic & Pacific (not King) | 1350-2100 | 8-13 |
| Tuna: Bluefin & Albacore | 1700 | 54-58 |
| Sardines: Atlantic & Pacific | 1100-1600 | 2 |
| Oysters: Pacific | 1500 | 2 |
| Trout: Freshwater | 1000-1100 | 11 |
| Tuna: White (Albacore) canned | 1000 | 40 |
| Mussels: Blue | 900 | NA* |
| Salmon: Pink & Sockeye | 700-900 | 2 |
| Squid | 750 | 11 |
| Pollock: Atlantic & Walleye | 600 | 6 |
| Marlin | 250-1030** | 69 |
| Crab: Blue, King, Snow, Queen & Dungeness | 200-550 | 9 |
| Tuna: Skipjack & Yellowfin | 150-350 | 31-49 |
| Flounder, Plaice & Sole (Flatfish) | 350 | 7 |
| Clams | 200-300 | <1*** |
| Tuna: Light canned | 150-300 | 13 |
| Catfish | 100-250 | 7 |
| Cod: Atlantic & Pacific | 200 | 14 |
| Scallops: Bay & Sea | 200 | 8 |
| Haddock & Hake | 200 | 2-5 |
| Lobster: American | 200 | 47 |
| Crayfish | 200 | 5 |
| Tilapia | 150 | 2 |
| Shrimp | 100 | <1*** |
| Orange Roughy | 42 | 80 |
| **Varieties That Should Not Be Consumed by Women Who are Pregnant or Breastfeeding or by Young Children** | | |
| Shark | 1250 | 151 |
| Tilefish: Gulf of Mexico | 1000 | 219 |
| Swordfish | 1000 | 147 |
| Mackerel: King | 450 | 110 |

Key: * *Not available. It is likely to be comparable to the levels in oysters & clams
**250 is the value for blue marlin and 1030 is the value for striped marlin
***Less than one

# What About Farmed Raised Fish?

For over a decade, there have been many warnings from environmental experts about the unsustainability of fish farms, also known as aquaculture. Conditions for farm-raised fish have sparked major controversy all over the world.

Farm-raised fish are often raised in such close confinement that some critics describe them as "swimming in their own feces." Their diets vary but often include artificial ingredients, antibiotics, GMO grains, and harmful chemicals that are passed on to humans when consumed. While the risks are certainly not clear, some experts believe that people who consume farmed salmon face a higher risk for retinal damage, cancer, antibiotic resistance, and potential reproductive damage.

Author of the bestselling book, *Grain Brain*, David Perlmutter, MD, provided five reasons in his book for avoiding farm-raised fish:

1. Farmed fish provides higher levels of inflammation-producing omega-6 fatty acids and lower levels of inflammation-fighting heart and brain healthy omega-3s. Dr. Perlmutter stated, "Inflammation is a key player in virtually all the medical issues you don't want to get including cancer, diabetes, arthritis, coronary artery disease and even Alzheimer's."

2. "Because of the crowded conditions in which farm-raised fish are raised, they are routinely treated with antibiotics to help prevent infection. Not only does this raise concern for residual antibiotics in the fish itself, but the use of antibiotics in this manner helps contribute to the ability of bacteria becoming more and more resistant to the very antibiotics we rely on to combat serious infectious diseases."

3. "Farm-raised fish may have as much as 20% less protein compared to wild fish."

4. "PCBs are cancer-causing chemicals that may exist in farm-raised salmon at a concentration 16 times higher than wild salmon, and the level of dioxin is also higher, by a factor of 11 fold."

5. "Finally, the notion that somehow fish farming is more 'sustainable' makes absolutely no sense at all. For every pound of salmon for instance, it takes 2-3 pounds of fish chow made from other fish like sardines, mackerel, anchovies, or herring. This needs to be factored into the equation as stocks of the fish used to sustain the fish farms are well on their way to becoming depleted."

Keep in mind that Atlantic salmon may sound like it's harvested in the Atlantic Ocean, however, it's almost always farm-raised. In contrast, salmon labeled "Alaskan" is not farmed. Alaska is extremely protective of their brand and they go to great lengths to ensure quality and sustainability. Because it's more expensive than farm-raised salmon, you can assume that the salmon served in restaurants is farm-raised, unless they tell specifically state otherwise. While there is some controversy about current practices in Alaska where fish are raised in hatcheries and released into the wild, this practice appears to be substantially different than that of "farmed-raised" fish, which are often fed GMO soy and corn and given antibiotics to treat and prevent sickness.

## Responsible Aquaculture?

While the majority of fish farms utilize poor farming practices resulting in water pollution and the overuse of chemicals and antibiotics, there is aquaculture that is committed to doing things responsibly.

The Aquaculture Stewardship Council (ASC) is an independent not-for-profit organization with a certification and labeling program that manages standards for responsible aquaculture. Products bearing the ASC label come from fish farms that have met the following seven standards:

1. Comprehensive legal compliance
2. Conservation of natural habitat and biodiversity
3. Conservation of water resources
4. Conservation of species diversity and wild population through prevention of escapes
5. Use of feed and other inputs that are sourced responsibly
6. Good animal health (no unnecessary use of antibiotics or chemicals)
7. Social responsibility for workers and communities impacted by farming (e.g. no child labor, health and safety of workers, freedom of association, community relations)

The ASC's logo gives consumers confidence that they are choosing seafood that comes from farms that limit their impact on the environment and community.

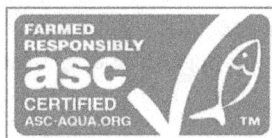

# Imported Seafood

Imported seafood is another area of major concern, since safety regulations may not be as stringent as those in place domestically. According to NOAA Fisheries (www.FishWatch.gov), a whopping 91 percent of seafood consumed in the United States is imported (about half of this is farm-raised). (31)

Consumers who eat imported seafood are exposed to whatever level of safety practices exist in the exporting country, including potential risks during processing, shipping and handling before it ever reaches the U.S.

There have been numerous recalls of contaminated imported seafood causing foodborne illness. One recent study in North Carolina revealed that one-quarter of seafood imported from China and Vietnam had detectable levels of formaldehyde, a known carcinogen commonly used as a medical disinfectant or embalming agent (www.foodsafetynews.com).

Fish from China, including tilapia has been found to contain leuco-malachite green, a chemical banned from use in aquaculture by the U.S. FDA in 1983 because of serious toxicity.

While you may not know if you're eating imported seafood at a restaurant, you can usually avoid it at the grocery store by asking the seafood department for the source or by checking the label on frozen seafood packaging.

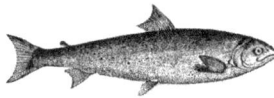

# How to Choose Your Fish

The following information was adapted from the Environmental Working Group's Good Seafood Guide and was intended to fill the gaps of the federal government's seafood guidance. It's designed to help consumers make better choices regarding the safest seafood to eat.

# Good Seafood Guide

| | | |
|---|---|---|
| **BEST BETS!**<br>Very High<br>Omega 3's<br>Low Mercury<br>Sustainable | WILD SALMON<br>SARDINES<br>MUSSELS<br>RAINBOW TROUT<br>ATLANTIC MACKEREL | One or two four-ounce servings a week of these fish have little mercury and optimum levels of omega-3 fatty acids for pregnant or nursing women and people with heart disease. |
| **GOOD CHOICES**<br>High Omega 3's<br>Low Mercury | OYSTERS<br>ANCHOVIES<br>POLLOCK/IMITATION CRAB<br>HERRING | These species have favorable concentrations of omega-3 fats. One four-ounce serving provides at least 25 percent of the weekly recommended omega-3 consumption. A pregnant woman of average weight could eat three four-ounce servings per week without ingesting too much mercury. These species do not necessarily come from sustainable sources. |
| **LOW MERCURY**<br>But Also Low<br>Omega-3's | SHRIMP<br>CATFISH<br>TILAPIA<br>CLAMS<br>SCALLOPS<br>PANGASIUS (BASA, SWAI, OR TRA) | These varieties can be healthy sources of protein and other nutrients, but an adult would have to eat five to 20 four-ounce portions to meet the omega-3 recommendation for pregnant women and people with heart disease. |
| **MERCURY RISKS ADD UP**<br>Pregnant Women<br>& Children Should<br>Limit or Avoid | CANNED LIGHT &<br>ALBACORE TUNA<br>HALIBUT<br>LOBSTER<br>MAHI MAHI<br>SEA BASS | These fish contain too much mercury to be part of the regular diet of pregnant women and children. How much you can safely eat depends on your age, weight and health status. Use EWG's Seafood Calculator to gauge how often you can eat them and to find healthier options. |
| **AVOID!**<br>Levels Too High To<br>Eat Regularly! | SHARK*<br>SWORDFISH*<br>TILEFISH*<br>KING MACKEREL*<br>MARLIN*<br>BLUEFIN & BIGEYE TUNA<br>STEAKS OR SUSHI**<br>ORANGE ROUGHY** | High-mercury seafood should never be eaten by pregnant women & children, according to EWG's analysis & federal government warnings. Everyone else should eat these species infrequently or not at all.<br><br>*FDA/EPA advisories recommend that pregnant women and children never eat these species.<br>** HIGH in mercury. |

# Meat & Poultry

Many Americans are aware of the major shift that is taking place today with regard to raising animals for food. We're seeing an increasing number of restaurants that are focused on meeting consumer demand for more sustainably raised meat and poultry. Companies are promising to support local farmers who utilize ethical practices by raising animals in a more natural, healthy environment, without the use of antibiotics or added growth hormones. These markets are booming due to the increasing demand from informed consumers who have learned the truth about the way livestock is being raised for food in the U.S.

Today's industrial agricultural practices have been labeled as "factory-farming," a negative term that is synonymous with extreme overcrowding of animals, serious health consequences, and major concern regarding the unethical treatment of animals. If you've watched any of the recent documentaries that expose factory-farming practices, then you've probably thought about becoming a vegetarian or vegan. It's not a pretty picture.

Let's take a quick look at what's been going on. When too many animals are crammed into ridiculously tight spaces with no room to move, you'd expect some serious health problems, right? This practice has led to the spread of disease, forcing the regular use of antibiotics to keep things under control. We all know that taking antibiotics on a daily basis would not be good for us. The American Academy of Pediatrics in collaboration with the Centers for Disease Control once again asked doctors to limit their use due to the serious concerns that overuse creates antibiotic resistance, putting children at greater risk for effective treatment of infections. Yet we're giving our children daily doses of antibiotics whenever they eat meat, poultry or dairy products that are treated with these substances.

As humans, we are what we eat, so wouldn't that apply to animals as well? We always have to think about the food chain to assess our own risk. Animals raised on factory-farms are being fed diets that will enhance their productivity and lower costs, including government-subsidized corn and soy, most of which are now genetically modified. They are fed hormones to fatten them up, and antibiotics to prevent the spread of nasty diseases caused by the filthy conditions associated with living in such close quarters. This represents the majority of meat Americans are eating and feeding to their children.

Fortunately, a growing number of ranchers have stopped these practices and have adopted more sustainable practices by sending their animals to pasture where they can live more natural lives and eat their native diet of grass rather than grains like corn, soy and other supplements that have been used to fatten them up. As a result, animals are growing at a more natural pace resulting in greater health, so there has been no need to use antibiotics.

Thankfully, it's not difficult to find organic, sustainably raised meat and poultry. Choosing quality over quantity is a wise approach for families who are budget-conscious. Organic grass-fed beef and organic free-range poultry are your best choices. (This also applies to eggs and dairy, by the way). Natural is not only healthier, but the best chefs won't settle for anything less.

## Organic Milk & Dairy Products

Organic milk, in general, comes from cows that eat only organic food that is not enhanced with antibiotics, hormones or other chemicals.

The USDA tightened their regulations for organic milk in February 2010, to include stricter rules about pasture access. Organic milk is now defined as milk from a cow that grazes on pasture at least four months out of each year, with at least 30 percent of the feed coming from grazing. In addition, ranchers must have a soil and water protection plan to protect quality.

Most organic milk in the U.S. is pasteurized, which has been shown to destroy vital nutrients. However, a new study has shown that organic homogenized/pasteurized and organic non-pastured milk may be superior to conventional milk. (32) Some of the significant differences between organic and conventional milk shown in the study include:

• Organic milk had 62% more omega-3 fats and contained 25% less omega-6 fats and than conventional milk. These higher ratios of Omega-6 fats to Omega-3 fats have been linked to many health problems.

The researchers noted:

*"Over the last century, intakes of omega-6 fatty acids in Western diets have dramatically increased, while omega-3 intakes have fallen. Resulting omega -6/3 intake ratios have risen to nutritionally undesirable levels, generally 10 to 15, compared to a possible optimal ratio near 2.3...We conclude that consumers have viable options to reduce average omega -6/3 intake ratios, thereby reducing or eliminating probable risk factors for a wide range of developmental and chronic health problems."*

31

- Pasture time may be responsible for the organic benefits. It's natural for cows to go to pasture and graze on grass, but today, cows that produce conventional milk are fed corn and other grains. This unnatural change affects their body composition including fat levels.

The researchers noted:

*"...milk from cows consuming significant amounts of grass and legume-based forages contains less [omega-6 fats] and higher concentrations of ALA, CLA, and the long-chain [omega-3s] EPA and DPA, compared to cows lacking routine access to pasture and fed substantial quantities of grains. In most countries, lactating cows on organically managed farms receive a significant portion of daily DMI [dry matter intake] from pasture and conserved, forage-based feeds, while cows on conventional farms receive much less. In the most recent U.S. government dairy sector survey, only 22% of cows had access to pasture, and for most of these, access was very limited in terms of average daily DMI."*

## Non-Organic Milk and rBST Growth Hormone

Have you noticed that most organic dairy products contain a statement on their label "from cows not treated with rBST"? Bovine somatotropin (BST) is a protein hormone that is naturally produced in a cow's pituitary glands. A recombinant version of rBST, also known as rBGH (recombinant Bovine Growth Hormone), was created by the agrichemical company, Monsanto, through the genetic engineering of E. coli bacteria. It is being marketed under the brand name "Posilac" for the purpose of increasing short-term milk production in cows. The use of this genetically modified growth hormone has spurred tremendous controversy worldwide and many countries have banned its use including Canada, Japan, Australia, New Zealand, and the 27 countries of the European Union.

## How Are the Animals Affected By rBST?

The possible side effects listed on Polisac's packaging include hoof disorders, reduced pregnancy rates, visibly abnormal milk, and the potential need for additional drug treatments (i.e. antibiotics) due to associated health problems such as mastitis. When cows are treated with rBST, they face a nearly 25% increase in the risk of mastitis, a 55% increased risk of lameness and a 40% reduction in fertility. (15)

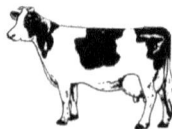

## How Does rBST Affect Milk Production?

Cows treated with rBST have also experienced elevated levels of insulin-like growth factor 1 (IGF-1), which can lead to increased IGF-1 in milk.[16] Many studies have noted a possible link between IGF-1 levels and an increased risk of cancer, particularly breast and prostate cancer. [17]

## Geez...Is Milk Even Healthy?

Milk has been a subject of much controversy in the health community for years, for reasons other than whether it's organic or conventional. Many health experts question the integrity of milk being touted as a health food in the first place.

A study, in *JAMA Pediatrics* [18] questions the scientific rationale for promoting milk consumption for both children and adults, and reconsiders the role of cow's milk in human nutrition. The authors stated:

*"Humans have no nutritional requirement for animal milk, an evolutionarily recent addition to diet. Anatomically modern humans presumably achieved adequate nutrition for millennia before domestication of dairy animals, and many populations throughout the world today consume little or no milk for biological reasons (lactase deficiency), lack of availability, or cultural preferences. Adequate dietary calcium for bone health, often cited as the primary rationale for high intakes of milk, can be obtained from other sources."*

Personally, our family uses very little dairy. If you are going to use milk and dairy products in your family, then by all means, choose organic if you want to avoid more toxins.

## Genetically Modified Organisms (GMOs)

Unlike traditional crossbreeding of crops and plant varieties, "genetically modified organisms" or GMOs are plants or animals that have been genetically engineered with DNA from bacteria, viruses, or other plants and animals, for the purpose of producing new combinations of genes and traits. These experimental combinations of genes taken from different species could never occur in nature or in traditional crossbreeding.

Despite FDA approval, GMOs have become one of the most fiercely debated topics around the world. There is question about the objectivity of this decision due to considerable profits associated with genetically engineered food.

Scientists around the world have been concerned about the long-term safety of GMOs as well as the uncertainty of their environmental impact. GMOs have been restricted or banned in more than 60 countries around the world, including Japan, Australia, and all countries in the European Union, yet in the U.S., even the labeling of GMOs is being debated.

**The American Academy of Environmental Medicine (AAEM)** has stated their concerns that, "Several animal studies indicate serious health risks associated with GM (genetically modified) food." According to the AAEM, "A 2008 study links GM corn with infertility, showing a significant decrease in offspring over time and significantly lower litter weight in mice fed GM corn. This study also noted that over 400 genes were found to be expressed differently in the mice fed GM corn. These are genes known to control protein synthesis and modification, cell signaling, cholesterol synthesis, and insulin regulation. Studies also show intestinal damage in animals fed GM foods, including proliferative cell growth and disruption of the intestinal immune system." The AAEM has recommended that physicians advise their patients to avoid GM foods.

## What are the Impacts of GMOs on the Environment?

The Non-GMO Project, a non-profit organization that is committed to educating consumers and providing verified non-GMO choices has concerns about the impact of GMOs on the environment, stating that,

"Over 80% of all GMOs grown worldwide are engineered for herbicide tolerance. As a result, use of toxic herbicides like Roundup™ has increased 15 times since GMOs were introduced. GMO crops are also responsible for the emergence of "super weeds" and "super bugs," which can only be killed with ever more toxic poisons like 2,4-D (a major ingredient in Agent Orange). GMOs are a direct extension of chemical agriculture, and are developed and sold by the world's biggest chemical companies. The long-term impacts of GMOs are unknown, and once released into the environment these novel organisms cannot be recalled."

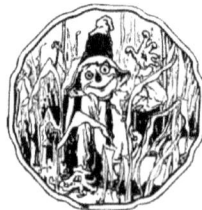

**High-Risk Crops include:**

1. **Alfalfa** (first planting 2011)
2. **Canola** (approx. 90% of U.S. crop)
3. **Corn** (approx. 88% of U.S. crop in 2011)
4. **Cotton** (approx. 90% of U.S. crop in 2011)
5. **Papaya** (most of Hawaiian crop; approximately 988 acres)
6. **Soy** (approx. 94% of U.S. crop in 2011)
7. **Sugar Beets** (approx. 95% of U.S. crop in 2010)
8. **Zucchini and Yellow Summer Squash** (approx. 25,000 acres)

(Source: Non-GMO Project Verified as of December 2011)

For more information and resources from the Non-GMO Project visit: www.nongmoproject.org. Look for this seal to ensure that a product is Non-GMO Verified:

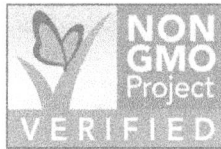

OMG – GMOs!

Does all of this focus on GMOs stress you out? It's easy to feel overwhelmed, so just start by taking baby steps. Check out the following "Non-GMO Tips" for suggestions on how to avoid GMOs and start to eliminate the sources you identify in your diet.

For the next couple of weeks, try paying closer attention to what you're eating and how you feel when you remove GMOs. You may be surprised by the difference in your mood, your energy level and even the effect these changes can have on your weight. Watch your kids and note the positive changes you see by removing GMOs from their diet. You may notice an improvement in their attention span. Remember this is a journey and every small step you take to reduce the toxins in your home can have a lifelong impact. ❤

# Non-GMO Tips

**Go Organic**
GMOs are prohibited by the USDA National Organic Standards, so buying organic is a great way to avoid them. Assume all non-organic corn, soy, cottonseed, and canola ingredients are GMO.

**Look For the Non-GMO-Verified Seal**
The USDA does not currently require GMO products to be labeled, so most companies won't tell us when foods contain GMOs. The Non-GMO Project seal is a trusted sign for consumers to identify if the product comes from best practices for GMO avoidance.

**Stay Away From Artificial Sweeteners**
Aspartame, which is manufactured by Monsanto, is made using genetically modified bacteria, according to sources cited in an article entitled "World's top sweetener is made with GM bacteria" (Independent, 1999).

**Choose Certified Organic Dairy Products**
Conventional dairy products come from cows treated with rBST or rBGH, a growth hormone that was created by Monsanto through the genetic engineering of E. coli bacteria. Organic dairy products are rBGH-free.

**Eat Lots of Fruits and Veggies**
Most fresh produce is non-GMO, with the exception of zucchini, yellow summer squash, edamame, sweet corn and papaya (from Hawaii or China) which are all considered high risk and are best avoided unless labeled "organic" or "non-GMO".

**Beware of Additives**
Five of the most common GMOs include corn, canola, soy, cotton and sugar beets, all of which often end up as additives in packaged foods (in the form of corn syrup, oil, sugar, flavoring agents or thickeners), so check ingredient labels carefully.

**Choose Wild-Caught Seafood**
Most farm-raised fish are not only considered unhealthy, but they are often fed with GMO feed.

**Limit Eating Out or Request Substitutions**
It's almost impossible to control the ingredients you're getting when you eat out, especially when they contain processed foods, soy sauce, cooking oil, or salad dressings, which often are hidden sources of GMOs. A good restaurant will often accommodate your request for substitutions such as cooking your fish with olive oil instead of canola oil, which will reduce your exposure to common GMO ingredients.

**Focus on fiber**
Most grains, seeds, nuts and beans are non-GMO.

Use the **Non-GMO Shopping Guide** from the Institute for Responsible Technology to help you choose healthier, non-GMO brands:
www.nongmoshoppingguide.com.

# 4 PURE CLEAN WATER

*"Water is the driving force of all nature."*
*Leonardo da Vinci*

Water is essential to sustain life and health, but if you're drinking your water straight out of the tap, you may want to think twice. Your tap water may actually be dirtier than it looks. According to a 3-year investigation by the Environmental Working Group (EWG.org) that tested the quality of drinking water around the country, Americans have a good reason to worry about drinking from the tap. Nationwide water utilities detected 316 chemicals of which more than half are unregulated and illegal in any amount.

Here are some helpful tips adapted from the "EWG Guide to Safe Drinking Water":

**1.   Bottled Water: Drink filtered tap water instead**.
You can read the bottle label, but you still won't know if the water is pure and natural or just processed, polluted, packaged tap water. EWG found 38 contaminants in 10 popular brands.

**2.   Tap Water: Learn what's in it.**
Tap water suppliers publish all their water quality tests. Bottled water companies don't. Read your annual tap water quality report. Look up your city's water in EWG's National Tap Water Atlas at (www.ewg.org/tap-water). Private well? Get it tested.

**3.   Filtered Tap Water: Drink it, cook with it.**
Choose a filter certified to remove contaminants found in your water: EWG Water Filter Buying Guide (EWG.org) Effectiveness varies - read the fine print.

Carbon filters (pitcher or tap-mounted) are affordable and reduce many common water contaminants, like lead and byproducts of the disinfection process used to treat municipal tap water.

Install a reverse osmosis (R/O) filter if you can afford it, to remove contaminants that carbon filters can't eliminate, like arsenic and perchlorate (rocket fuel). This is the most effective water purification system.

**4.  Filters: Change them.**
Change your water filters on time. Old filters aren't safe – they harbor bacteria and let contaminants through. (Don't forget the one in your refrigerator, if you have that feature!)

**5.  On the Go: Carry water in safe containers.**
Hard plastic bottles (#7 plastic) can leach a harmful plastics chemical called bisphenol A (BPA) into water. Carry stainless steel or other BPA-free bottles. Don't reuse bottled water bottles. The plastic can harbor bacteria and break down to release plastic chemicals.

**6.  While Pregnant: Stay hydrated with safe water.**
It's especially important for women to drink plenty of water during pregnancy. Follow all the tips above, and take your doctor's advice on how much to drink.

**7.  Infants: Use safe water for formula.**
Use filtered tap water for your baby's formula. If your water is not fluoridated, you can use a carbon filter. If it is, use a reverse osmosis filter to remove the fluoride, because fluoridated water can damage an infant's developing teeth. If you choose bottled water for your infant, make sure it's fluoride-free.
Learn more at EWG Baby Guide (www.EWG.org).

**8.  Breathe Easy: Use a whole house water filter.**
For extra protection, a whole house carbon filter will remove contaminants from steamy vapors you and your family inhale while showering and washing dishes. Effectiveness varies widely – call the manufacturer for details.

## How to Choose a Water Filter

For guidance on the best type of water filter for your home, visit the EWG's Water Filter Buying Guide @ EWG.org.

Investing in water filtration is an important part of avoiding the chemicals in your water supply. Your family will even taste the difference. Filtering water at home not only can remove those harmful contaminants, it will save you a lot of money over buying plastic water bottles. Work toward filtering the water your family bathes in to reduce chlorine and other chemical exposure. Even your hair and skin will thank you. ❤

# 5 BREATHE CLEAN

We tend to think of air pollution as being outside, like smog or ozone. But a growing body of scientific evidence indicates that the air in our home is often more seriously polluted than the air outside. The EPA estimates that we spend as much as 90% of our time indoors which is a big deal, especially for those who are more at risk, our children. (33)

The National Safety Council reports that children breathe in 50 percent more air per pound of body weight than adults do. Environmental Protection Agency (EPA) studies have found that pollution levels inside our homes can be two to five times higher than outdoors and even as high as 100 times higher than outdoors after some activities. (33)

## Sources of Indoor Pollution

Every home has countless sources of indoor air pollution. Obvious ones include cleaning products, pesticides and chemicals. Less obvious are the things that create off-gassing, the release of noxious gases from sources such as building materials, furniture, carpet, shower curtains, and pressed wood.

## Asthma Prevention

Energy efficient measures to keep our heat and air conditioning inside have created airtight homes that trap pollutants inside as well. According to a recent study, published in the American Journal of Respiratory and Critical Care Medicine, 65% of asthma cases among elementary school-age children could be prevented by controlling exposure to indoor allergens and environmental tobacco smoke (ETS). (34) They also concluded that by controlling biological contaminants such as pet dander, dust mites and cat allergens, asthma cases could be reduced by 55 to 60%. There's plenty we can do to improve the air quality in our homes.

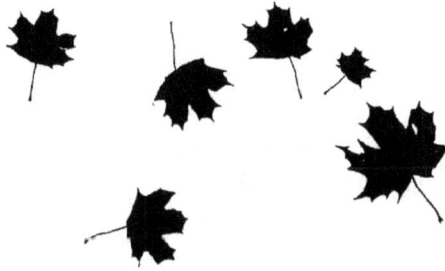

# 12 Tips To Help You Breathe Easier

### 1. Use Low-VOC Paints

Paints can emit trace amounts of gases for months, even after they have fully dried and there is no longer an odor. These gases, called VOCs, or volatile organic compounds, can contain highly toxic chemicals such as formaldehyde and acetaldehyde. With so much demand for "green" products today, most major paint brands carry a line of "low-VOC" products. These are your best choices. Always remember to open windows and use exhaust fans while painting or using products with chemicals. Never leave open paint containers indoors. Because children are much more susceptible to harm due to their size, it's always best to keep them away from these projects, especially those with asthma.

### 2. Don't Allow Smoking Indoors

According to the Surgeon General, there is no safe level of secondhand smoke. Protect your family and never allow anyone to smoke in your home.

### 3. Install a Carbon Monoxide Detector

Each year, an average of 500 hundred people die from accidental carbon monoxide poisoning and thousands of others end up in the emergency room due to exposure to this odorless gas. It may appear that someone has the flu, however consider carbon monoxide poisoning when more than one member of your family has symptoms, including your pets. If you feel better when away from home, then carbon monoxide may be the problem.

The best way to protect your family from this silent killer is to install a carbon monoxide detector near your bedrooms. If you have any fuel-burning appliances, it's important to have them professionally inspected every year.

### 4.  Test for Radon

Radon is an invisible but lethal killer that could be in your home. It's actually the primary cause of lung cancer in nonsmokers and the second-leading cause of lung cancer, period.  Radon is an odorless, invisible gas that naturally occurs in soil and rock.  Testing is easy and inexpensive and can save your life.  To learn how to test for radon, visit this EPA website: epa.gov/radon/radontest.html.

### 5.  Keep Things Dry

Dampness in your home promotes a breeding ground for dangerous mold and mildew.  Inspect your home regularly for any evidence of water, including a wet ceiling, leaking roof, damp basement or any cracks or leaks around the foundation.  Be sure to re-route water to keep it away from your home's foundation and fix problems promptly to prevent unhealthy toxins from growing.  If moisture is present due to humidity, consider a dehumidifier or run the air conditioner, and be sure to keep them clean to prevent the spread of airborne allergens.  Mold and mildew are major triggers of respiratory problems such as asthma, coughing, and wheezing.

### 6.  Be Aware of the Dangers of Candles

According to a study performed at South Carolina State University (35), the chemicals emitted by paraffin candles are linked to cancer, birth defects, and respiratory ailments such as asthma, particularly when burned in unventilated areas.  The most common and inexpensive candles are made of paraffin wax, a petroleum bi-product.  Paraffin candles emit black soot that is chemically similar to the poisonous chemicals in diesel exhaust.

## Scented Candles

Be wary of scented candles because the added scents are often synthetic chemicals that can cause cancer and exacerbate allergies and asthma.  Just because a candle is made from a natural wax like soy doesn't mean that the fragrance is safe.

Marketers know all the buzzwords that consumers are looking for today, so it's important to make sure you know what you're getting.

Scented candles have long been known to be a trigger for migraine headaches.  Babies and children are particularly at risk for reactions, especially those with respiratory issues.

As someone who is extremely sensitive to chemical scents, I can tell you that it's very awkward to be a guest in someone's home when they are burning a scented candle (that they feel is creating a special ambiance). Be sensitive to your guests and protect your family by avoiding scented candles.

## Lead Wicks

For many years, scented candles on the market contained lead-core wicks. Scented oils can soften wax, so manufacturers used lead to make the wicks firmer. A lead-core wick emits 5 times the hazardous limit of lead for children and has been linked to serious health problems including hormone disruption, behavioral problems and learning disabilities. Although lead wicks were banned in 2003, some people still have them in their homes either because they were purchased years ago, or because the candles were imported from China or Hong Kong where these regulations do not apply.

Young children and unborn babies are particularly at risk because even small amounts of lead can cause a loss in I.Q. in addition to learning disabilities and behavior problems. Pregnant women should be especially wary of any lead exposure since the placenta offers no barrier to lead and exposure can result in miscarriage or brain and nervous system damage to a fetus. **If you're not sure whether your candle contains a lead-core wick, you can perform the simple test below.**

---

**Simple Lead Wick Test**

To determine if a candle has a lead wick, perform these simple steps:

1. For candles that have not been burned, rub the tip of the wick on a piece of white paper. If it leaves a gray mark similar to a pencil, the wick contains a lead core.

2. For candles that have been burned, simply look at the tip of the wick and you can see the metal core. You can peel back the cotton if it's not visible.

3. Always look for a "lead-free" label when buying a candle.

4. If you have a lead wick candle, throw it out.

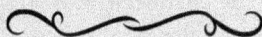

---

**Candle Recommendations:**

- Choose non-toxic, unscented candles made from unbleached beeswax or soy. These candles produced no toxic chemicals in the aforementioned study.

- Never buy candles made from paraffin—a petroleum bi-product that releases soot and toxic chemicals when burned.

- Don't be fooled by marketing. A scented soy candle may be non-toxic, however, if you're not sure, don't buy it. Synthetic chemical scents can cause cancer.

- Check your wicks to be sure they have no metal core since that would indicate they contain lead, a very serious toxin. Although lead wicks were banned in 2003, you may still have them in your home. Check the wicks of older candles as well as those that may be imported using the simple lead test. Look for those labeled as "lead-free".

- Because scented candles are a common trigger for headaches and asthma symptoms, consider buying unscented candles. For healthier scents in your home, try using pure essential oils for aromatherapy. These are non-toxic and can be very relaxing, however, keep in mind that even pure essential oils can be irritating to some people with sensitivities.

- Purchase candles from suppliers who are committed to provide non-toxic, pure products.

## Flameless Alternatives

If you'd like to avoid candles completely, there are now some very realistic flameless candles that are battery powered (some with timers). Some of these are so realistic that someone may try to blow them out. Quality ones are not cheap, but there are trade-offs, including not having to replace them as quickly as you would a traditional candle. The technology has come a long way with some amazing 3D flames. I purchased a flameless candle for my daughter, since I don't allow her to burn anything in her room. She loves it and feels that it creates the same relaxing atmosphere of a traditional candle. I highly recommend that you buy an unscented flameless candle or you will be bringing more irritating toxic chemicals into your home.

## 7. Beware of Dry Cleaning Chemicals

Many people don't realize that dry cleaning solvents are extremely toxic and pose major health and environmental concerns. According to the EPA, a predominant chemical solvent used in dry cleaning, PERC (perchloroethylene), is considered a human health hazard affecting reproduction and development, kidneys, liver, and immune and hemotologic systems.

PERC has been shown to cause cancer in rats and mice when they ingest or inhale it. In fact, studies of workers in the dry cleaning industry have demonstrated elevated risks of certain cancers (bladder, non-Hodgkin's lymphoma and multiple myeloma).

Despite the name, dry cleaning is actually not a dry process. Clothing is submerged into liquid PERC for cleaning and it readily evaporates into the air. It lingers in dry-cleaned clothing fibers and is slowly released into your home and car. Since you're wearing clothing that has been submerged in it, you're also likely to be absorbing it through skin with direct contact.

Symptoms from exposure can include dizziness, fatigue, headaches, confusion, nausea, skin, lung, eye, and mucus membrane irritation.

PERC is also used in products such as adhesives, correction fluid, wood cleaners and spot removers. It's found in many carpet cleaners, which like dry cleaners, use it to remove stains. Residues from dry-cleaned carpets can linger on the carpet fibers and actually attract more dirt. When cleaning carpets, it's best to use steam cleaners without chemicals.

PERC is found is in many automobile-cleaning products because of its ability to cut through grease. To avoid exposure, choose non-toxic cleaners like vinegar or a trusted non-toxic cleaner.

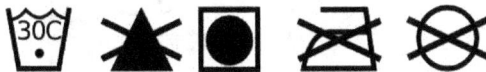

# Dry Cleaning Tips

- If clothing has been dry-cleaned using PERC, hang items outdoors to air out before bringing them inside to prevent chemicals from entering your home.

- Choose to use a non-toxic alternative to traditional dry cleaning. Here are some options you may want to consider:

- Look for "wet-cleaning," an alternative form of washing and drying that is safe for most clothing.

  - ✓ The National Clearinghouse for Wet Cleaners provides resources to help you locate one in your area: http://www.professionalwetcleaning.com.

  - ✓ CO2 cleaning, which uses liquid carbon dioxide to clean clothes is another safe alternative.

  - ✓ Consider hand-washing your garments in cold water. Many items, such as wool, rayon, and silk can be safely hand-washed even when the label says "Dry Clean" (not "Dry Clean ONLY").

- Some non-PERC dry-cleaners use alternatives that are sometimes called "hydrocarbon" treatments. Be aware that these are also considered toxic.

## 8.  Watch Out for Formaldehyde

Formaldehyde is a chemical that is used in thousands of home products, including bonding agents, disinfectants, adhesives, particleboard, plywood, paneling, pressed-wood products, and foam insulation. It has a strong pickle-like odor.  It is also found in some synthetic fabrics, including permanent press, as well as cosmetics, shampoos, and keratin hair straighteners.

Formaldehyde is classified as a volatile organic compound (VOC), a classification of chemicals that becomes a gas at room temperature. Products containing formaldehyde will release the gas into the air, a process known as "off-gassing."

Because formaldehyde is a product of combustion, burning materials such as natural gas, wood, gasoline, or tobacco will release formaldehyde gas.

The most common symptoms related to formaldehyde exposure are eye, nose and throat irritation, coughing, headaches, dizziness, and nausea. Anyone with asthma may be more sensitive to formaldehyde.

The Environmental Protection Agency (EPA) has listed formaldehyde as a "probable human carcinogen."

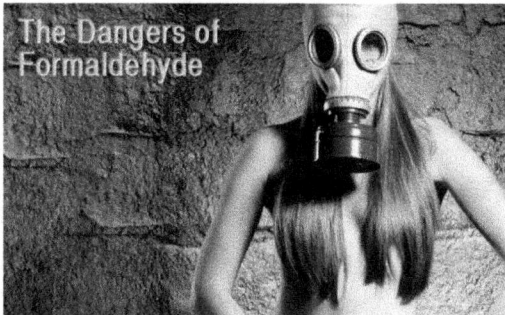

Source: http://www.kerapure.com/the-dangers-of-formaldehyde/

### 9. Avoid Pesticides

Pesticide chemicals are designed to kill—they are toxic to our families and our pets and damage our environment. Because many of us go crazy when we spot a creepy bug crawling in our home, why not decide in advance how we want to deal with these pests so we avoid over-reacting with chemicals. There are many non-toxic options that can be very effective at controlling pests.

## Integrated Pest Management

Today many experts are recommending that we take a step back from conventional pest control and focus on Integrated Pest Management (IPM), a common sense approach to managing the pests in our lives. IPM utilizes biological, cultural, and mechanical methods to control pests, and resorts to toxic pesticides only as a last resort. It is an environmentally sensitive and economically sound pest control approach that can result in healthier pest management.

There are basically 4 steps to IPM:

1. Set Action Thresholds: It's important to set a threshold for taking action before we have a problem with pests. For example, when you see ants crawling all over your kitchen countertop, it's probably not necessary to call a pest control company. However when you see termites swarming, which pose an economic threat to your home, immediate action may be required. Deciding these thresholds in advance will help you to make better decisions.

2. Monitor and Identify Pests: Many pests are innocuous and even beneficial, especially in our gardens (i.e. spiders & lady bugs). When becoming a Master Gardener, I was surprised to learn that only 3% of insects in a garden are actually harmful. IPM suggested that you monitor and identify pests accurately so that you can make the best decisions on how to control them. Monitoring and identification reduces the possibility that pesticides will be used when they are not really needed, and if they cannot be avoided, that the best choices will be made.

3. Prevention: Your first line of defense is always prevention when it comes to keeping pests out of your home, off of your lawn, and out of your garden.

4. Control: Once monitoring, identification, and action thresholds indicate that pest control is required, and preventive methods are no longer effective or available, IPM programs then evaluate the proper control method both for effectiveness and risk. Effective, less *risky* pest controls should always be chosen before resorting to toxic ones.

The EPA has issued a publication with tips for controlling pests in your home in a safe, non-toxic way. (24) Here are some of their suggestions:

1) Starve Them Out
2) Dry Them Out
3) Keep Them Out

---

## TIPS TO STARVE THEM OUT!

Pests will eat just about anything, but they might leave you alone if they don't have easy access to food:

- Seal up boxes and bags of food. Roaches love cardboard boxes and can climb into these items with ease.

- Store open food in sealed bags or containers, such as cereal, flour, or sugar (preferably glass to reduce plastics).

- Immediately clean up spills and leftover crumbs. Pests love free food left out in the open. Always clean up before bed.

- Don't walk around the house while eating. Meals and snacks eaten at a table are easier to control.

- Clean dirty dishes right away. Pests want whatever is left of your meals. Avoid leaving dirty dishes in sink, especially overnight.

- Keep a tight lid on trash, and empty it often. It may be trash to you, but pests see it as dinner. Place trashcans far away from a back door entrance.

- Don't leave pet food out overnight. Food can stir up pests' appetites. Roaches love to drink from a dog bowl.

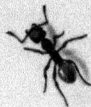

## TIPS TO DRY THEM OUT

Although roaches can live up to one month without food; without water roaches can die in a week's time:

- Always drain dishwater from a sink. Because roaches can swim, a sink full of water might become the site of a roach pool party.

- Wipe water and other spilled liquids off the counter as soon as you first see it. Puddles are roach magnets.

- Fix or report leaky faucets, radiators, dishwashers, and washing machines to a building manager.

- Empty excess water in flowerpots and plant stands. A drop of water can be all a roach needs to feel satisfied.

## TIPS TO KEEP THEM OUT!

By keeping roaches and rodents out of your home, you can prevent them from ever becoming a problem. Rodents spend most of their lives hiding. They love cracks, and can squeeze just about anywhere. Think smart, and they can't move in on you:

- Seal cracks and openings along baseboards, behind sinks, and around pipes and windows.

- Repair holes in door and window screens to prevent insects and other pests from entering a home.

- Check boxes and bags for roaches before bringing them into a home. They will multiply.

- Clean up clutter, including stacks of newspapers, paper bags, and cardboard boxes. These make good hiding places for pests.

- Set traps to control rats and mice. If you use baits, make sure they are in a tamper-resistant bait station made of durable plastic or metal, and place in an area where children and pets cannot touch them.

## 10. Ventilate Your Bathrooms

Where there is moisture, there is a potential for mold to grow. Bathrooms are already considered to be breeding grounds for germs, but they pose additional risks when moisture is a factor. Fans can be an effective way to help reduce mold growth by pulling out moisture. Use common sense if you smell any mold or see water spots.

## 11. Ventilate Your Kitchen

Cooking is another big source of indoor air pollution, especially when you cook on a gas stove (which I prefer). One study showed that cooking a single meal on a gas stove can produce levels of nitrogen dioxide that are considered unsafe to breath according to EPA standards. Be sure your kitchen stove is well ventilated to the outside or open a window whenever you cook. This is especially important when you use the self-cleaning setting on your oven.

## 12. Reduce Carpeting

Carpet can be a breeding ground for unhealthy particles, dust mites, pet dander, and can even off-gas chemicals. Many allergists recommend removing carpet in homes, particularly when children suffer with asthma or allergies, since this will significantly reduce irritating pollutants. If you do have carpets, consider investing in a vacuum cleaner that does not allow particulates back in the air, such as a HEPA (high efficiency particle air). Vacuuming itself can stir up airborne particles. Less toxic alternatives to carpet include hard surface flooring made of wood, tile or cork. As carpet wears out, consider replacing it with wood or another hard surface.

Awareness is our best friend when it comes to keeping our homes safe from toxic chemicals. Even with all the hidden sources of exposure, we can make a difference in the quality of the air we breathe simply by opening our windows more often and avoiding some of the most common forms of indoor air pollution. Take a deep breath and smile. ♥

# 6 CLEAN HOME

The typical American home is filled with cleaning products containing toxic chemicals that have been linked to asthma, cancer, hormone disruption, damage to reproductive organs, neurotoxicity, and much more.

One 15-year study presented at the Toronto Indoor Air Conference (36) reported that women who work at home have a 54% higher death rate from cancer than those who work away from home. The study concluded that this was a direct result of the much higher exposure to toxic chemicals that are commonly found in household products. Consider what these same chemicals can do to our children who inhale far more of them than an adult due to their size.

The American Academy of Pediatrics called for a major overhaul of the 35-year-old federal law that governs toxic chemicals, stating that it fails to safeguard children and pregnant women. In reference to this law, they stated the following, "It is widely recognized to have been ineffective in protecting children, pregnant women and the general population from hazardous chemicals in the marketplace."

The Academy pointed out in their policy statement that children face greater risks because they eat, drink, and breathe more pound for pound than adults, and they spend more time on the floor or the ground than adults, a possible source of exposure.

The very things we use to clean our homes are the primary sources of indoor air pollution that we are exposing our families to every day.

# Greenwashing

Despite marketing claims, many "green" products have been found to contain harmful ingredients. Because of the increasing market demand for non-toxic products that are kind to the environment and safer for humans, consumers are finding it more difficult than ever to determine which companies are truly dedicated to being green and walking the talk. The term "greenwashing" is used to describe companies that are just pretending to make a difference so that we'll buy their products, something we're seeing a lot of these days.

Another reason things are getting trickier for consumers is because many ingredients do not even have to be listed on the label, making it even more difficult to discern the dangers. There is continuous lobbying going on with manufacturers seeking government exemption from listing ingredients used in proprietary formulations, saying it's a trade secret. It's no surprise that many of these non-disclosed ingredients are toxic. The more informed we are as consumers, the harder manufacturers have to work to protect their interests.

Women's Voices for the Earth (WVE), a nonprofit consumer advocate group, commissioned an independent laboratory to test twenty popular cleaning products for hidden toxic chemicals from five top companies: Clorox, Procter & Gamble, Reckitt Benckiser, SC Johnson and Son, and Sunshine Makers (Simple Green). The report "Dirty Secrets: What's Hiding In Your Cleaning Products?" includes testing on all-purpose cleaners, laundry detergents, dryer sheets, air fresheners, disinfectant sprays, and furniture polish and exposes toxic chemicals that companies are keeping secret from consumers.

A copy of the report, Dirty Secrets can be found at: www.womensvoices.org.

> *Integrity is doing the right thing,*
> *even when no one is watching.*
> *C.S. Lewis*

# What's Under Your Sink?

**Ammonia**
Irritating to eyes and mucous membranes. Can cause breathing difficulty, wheezing, chest pains, pulmonary edema, and skin burns. High exposure can lead to blindness, lung damage, heart attack, or death.

**Carpet Cleaners**
Extremely toxic to children. The fumes given off by carpet cleaners can cause cancer and liver damage.

**Chlorine** The chemical most frequently involved in household poisonings and a potent pollutant. May cause reproductive, endocrine, and immune system disorders.

**Degreasers** May contain petroleum distillates and butyl cellosolve, which can damage lung tissues and dissolve fatty tissue surrounding nerve cells.

**Drain Cleaners** One of the most hazardous products in the home. Can contain lye, which is a strong caustic substance that causes severe corrosive damage to eyes, skin, mouth, and stomach. Can be fatal if swallowed.

**Oven Cleaners** One of the most dangerous cleaning products. Can cause severe damage to eyes, skin, mouth, and throat.

**Scouring Cleansers** May contain butyl cellosolve, a petroleum-based solvent that can irritate mucous membranes and cause liver and kidney damage.

**Toilet Bowl Cleaners** One of the most dangerous cleaning products. Can contain chlorine and hydrochloric acid. Harmful to health simply by breathing during use.

**Tub and Tile Cleaners** Can contain chlorine and may contribute to the formation of organochlorines, a dangerous class of compounds that can cause reproductive, endocrine, and immune system disorders.

# Laundry

Did you know that chemicals in your laundry soap can make you feel more fatigued and can leave you feeling short of breath? Laundry soaps can contain many toxic chemicals that stay in the fibers of your clothing, so they are inhaled and absorbed through the skin all day and night.

Some of the chemicals found in popular laundry products include:
- **Phenols** have been known to harm the lungs, kidneys, liver, and heart.
- **Artificial fragrances** have been linked to cancer and asthma. These can also affect our sense of smell.
- **1-4 dioxane** is a solvent that has been linked to kidney and liver damage.

Short-term inhalation has been shown to cause vertigo, headaches, drowsiness, anorexia, and irritation to the eyes, throat, nose, and lungs. All of these chemicals can cause skin rashes and itching and can irritate the respiratory system.

My son had a chronic skin rash that started at a very early age. When I started using a more natural laundry detergent, his rash cleared up immediately. The rash re-occurred when he went off to college and used a different detergent, and once again, it cleared up when he stopped using it. This appears to be a common problem for many children, especially those with allergies and skin sensitivities.

## Tips for Choosing Non-Toxic Cleaners

### 1. Make Your Own Cleaners

Some people prefer to make their own non-toxic cleaners. Here are some great resources that provide simple "recipes" for cleaning:

- Non-Toxic DIY Recipes from the WVE website: www.womensvoices.org/avoid-toxic-chemicals/diy-recipes/.

- Greatist.com is a website that also offers some excellent suggestions for making your own non-toxic cleaners.

## 2. Find Brands You Can Trust

The Environmental Working Group (EWG) published an excellent resource: "Guide to Healthy Cleaning" that is available on their website (EWG.org). There are many less toxic brands on the market today. Some work and some do not (in my opinion). Some are truly green, while others are not, but say they are.

One of the best ways to protect your family from toxic chemicals is to become an informed, smart shopper. No one cares more about protecting your children than you do. ♥

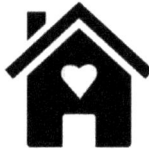

*On a personal note…after years of extensive research, I found a company that I can trust, Shaklee. I appreciate all that they do to ensure product integrity, purity, and safety, so that I can feel confident using their products in our home. This humble company has quietly led the way in environmental stewardship and support of social causes. While I've been disappointed in the performance of many "green" products on the market, I love that these perform exceptionally well, save lots of money & have a 100% guarantee, so I feel great about sharing them with you. xo*

# 7 CHEMICALS ABSORBED THROUGH OUR SKIN

*"Take care of your body. It's the only place you have to live." Jim Rohn*

The average woman uses 12 personal care products each day, and the average man uses 6 a day, exposing themselves to over 126 unique chemical ingredients, according to a consumer survey from the Environmental Working Group. Most of us have gone through this ritual for so long that we don't give it much thought, but maybe we should.

In a recent talk given to the Harvard School of Public Health (HSPH) entitled "Toxic Trespass: Harmful & Untested Chemicals in Everyday Products," Mia Davis, head of health and safety for a personal care product company stated, "The lipstick we wear, the food we eat, and the soap we use to clean our children's hands often contain harmful chemicals. The load adds up quickly day after day. And as we swallow, breathe in, and lather up, toxins entering our bodies may have lasting impact."

It's probably no surprise that so many experts believe that these chemicals are linked to the rising rates in asthma, breast cancer, reproductive problems, autism, and other health issues.

## Who is Responsible for Substantiating the Safety of Cosmetics?

Many chemicals in personal care products have little if any testing for safety, and there is a growing concern that all of these different chemicals are accumulating in our bodies over time and interacting in ways that may be extremely dangerous to our health.

The FDA states on their website that "Companies and individuals who manufacture or market cosmetics have a legal responsibility to ensure the safety of their products. Neither the law nor FDA regulations require specific tests to demonstrate the safety of individual products or ingredients. The law also does not require cosmetic companies to share their safety information with the FDA." In other words, the companies who produce the cosmetics are responsible for protecting consumers. That's reassuring.

With the exception of certain color additives and a handful of prohibited substances, cosmetic companies are allowed to use any raw ingredient they choose, including many chemicals that do not require government review or approval. In contrast, the European Union has banned over a 1000 different ingredients for cosmetic use.

Because there is a lack of FDA regulation over cosmetics in the U.S., the FDA has authorized the cosmetics industry to police itself through their own "Cosmetic Ingredient Review" panel. Only 11 ingredients/chemical groups have been declared unsafe during the past 30 years since its establishment and their recommendations to restrict ingredients are not binding on cosmetic companies. (37)

Many consumers believe that when they apply cosmetics to their skin, they do not get into their body, and if they do, the amounts are not significant enough for concern. The fact is that the chemicals in cosmetics can enter our bodies through sprays and powders that we breath, lotions that are applied to our skin, and by swallowing them when they are on the lips. Studies have found that many dangerous ingredients, including paraben preservatives, phthalate plasticizers, pesticide triclosan, synthetic musks and sunscreen ingredients are polluting the bodies of most children, women and men, and many of these chemicals are hormone disruptors. (19)

Numerous studies have linked health problems including damage to sperm, feminization of male reproductive organs, and low birth weight of girls, to exposure to chemicals found in common fragrance and sunscreen ingredients. (20)

Another common belief among consumers is that products labeled as "hypoallergenic" are safer choices. This type of terminology is not required to be backed up by companies, even for children's products. According to the FDA, the terms "hypoallergenic" and "natural" can mean anything, yet from a marketing standpoint, they are generally considered to be safer by consumers.

## Natural or Organic Labeling

Products labeled as natural or organic may contain synthetic chemicals, including petrochemicals. They are currently only required to contain 10% organic ingredients by weight or volume. (38) Even truly organic ingredients are not always risk-free.

The FDA currently has no authority to recall a cosmetic that causes injury, rather, they rely on companies to voluntarily report any cosmetic-related injuries (FDA 2005).

## Trade Secrets

Companies are allowed to leave some chemical ingredients off their product labels, including trade secrets, fragrance components and nanomaterials and fragrances. Over 3100 stock chemicals are not required to be listed. (39) Studies performed on these same fragrance ingredients have revealed 14 hidden compounds per formulation, including ingredients linked to sperm damage and hormone disruption. (EWG & CSC 2010)

While it's impossible to escape these chemicals completely, we can significantly reduce our exposure by making some simple, more informed choices. Several non-profit organizations including the Environmental Working Group (EWG) and Healthy Child, Healthy World offer excellent consumer resources to help us choose safer products for our families. By educating our children and teaching them to read labels, we can empower them to make better decisions.

We're seeing greater legislative movement in the direction of regulating the safety of products that are marketed to consumers, including **The Cosmetics and Personal Care Products Act of 2013** (H.R. 1385), which was introduced on March 21, 2013. It was designed to give the U.S. Food and Drug Administration authority to ensure that personal care products are free of harmful ingredients and that ingredients are fully disclosed.

## Hair Coloring Treatments

Hair coloring, including highlights and lowlights, has become a common practice among women today, whether or not you even have gray hair to cover. These choices are very personal and my goal is merely to present the concerns around toxicity and some options available to facilitate making more informed decisions with regard to your health.

Let me start by saying that pregnant women are generally cautioned by their obstetricians to avoid hair dyes, especially during their first trimester, and often beyond. There are good reasons for this caution, so if you are pregnant or considering becoming pregnant, you may want to look more closely at the associated risks.

Here are some facts about hair dye toxicity:

- The Environmental Working Group tested hair dye products and found that 69% may pose cancer risks.
- The National Cancer Institute reported in 1994 that dark hair dyes used over long periods of time appear to increase the risk of certain cancers such as non-Hodgkin's lymphoma and multiple myeloma.
- The International Journal of Cancer featured a study in 2001 stating that those who use permanent hair dye are twice as likely to develop bladder cancer as those who don't dye their hair.
- Hair dye is not regulated by the FDA or any other agency.

Many conventional hair dyes contain hazardous chemicals that should be avoided, if possible, including:

- Ammonia
- Coal Tar (FDA warning 1993 re: cancer risk)
- Lead
- Peroxide
- PPDs (para-phenylenediamines)- chemicals that create color, believed to be carcinogenic
- Resorcinol
- Toluene

## At-Home Hair Dyes

There's really no such thing as "organic" hair dyes, despite marketing claims. There are conventional dyes that contain many synthetic chemicals and there are more natural choices like vegetable-based dyes and henna. Most of the more natural choices still contain questionable ingredients, however, the at-home natural dyes appear to be significantly less risky than the conventional ones. The majority of these dyes are made in Europe, which is interesting since the European Commission banned 22 hair dye chemicals in 2006 that were potentially linked to bladder cancer.

Here is a list of the 22 chemicals banned in Europe. If you're concerned about the toxicity level of your hair coloring, then check to see if the products you are using contain any of these chemicals. If they do, then you may want to look for something else:

- 6-Methoxy-2,3-Pyridinediamine
- 2,3 Naphthalenediol
- 2,4-Diaminodiphenylamine
- 2,6-Bis(2-Hydroxyethoxy)-3,5-Pyridinediamine
- 2-Methoxymethyl-p-Aminophenol
- 4,5-Diamino-1-Methylpyrazole
- 4,5-Diamino-1-((4-Chlorophenyl)Methyl)-1H-Pyrazole Sulfate
- 4-Chloro-2-Aminophenol
- 4-Hydroxyindole
- 4-Methoxytoluene-2,5-Diamine
- 5-Amino-4-Fluoro-2-Methylphenol Sulfate
- N,N-Diethyl-m-Aminophenol
- N,N-Dimethyl-2,6-Pyridinediamine
- N-Cyclopentyl-m-Aminophenol
- N-(2-Methoxyethyl)-p-phenylenediamine
- 2,4-Diamino-5-methylphenetol
- 1,7-Naphthalenediol
- 3,4-Diaminobenzoic acid
- 2-Aminomethyl-p-aminophenol
- Solvent Red 1 (CI 12150)
- Acid Orange 24 (CI 20170)
- Acid Red 73 (CI 27290)

You can find the more natural hair dyes that you can apply at home in many health food stores and natural grocery store chains such as Whole Foods. If you've never used them, it may be prudent to discuss your options with knowledgeable staff to be sure you get the best results. Whether you can achieve the outcome you desire with a more natural product is for you to decide.

The EWG has evaluated many of the at-home dyes for safety and results are posted on their "Skin Deep" database at www.EWG.org/skindeep.

## Salon Hair Coloring

If you prefer to go to a salon for professional hair coloring, it turns out there may be some better options than others. Aveda is an option that claims to be more naturally derived than conventional salon brands used.

Here's what Annie Berthold Bond, author of "Better Basics for the Home: Simple Solutions for Less Toxic Living" had to say about Aveda:

"Salon brands of hair dye are almost all 100% synthetic and petroleum-based. The dyes are usually the controversial oxidative dyes. Aveda uses oxidative dyes like the rest of the industry (albeit in a small percentage), because so far there are no plant formulas that can provide consistent, long-lasting dyes. Oxidative dyes make up the 1% to 3% synthetic ingredients of the Aveda formulations. Oxidative dyes have no pre-existing colors until they are combined and joined with oxidizing ingredients. Most dyes use a synthetic to do this, but Aveda did research into essential oils and plant extracts, and they found and patented a process to oxidize the dye using green tea extract. Not only is the end process less petroleum-based, the result is more natural looking. The common base formulas for dyes are petrochemical solvents, and in this process Aveda has substituted protective and lubricating plant oils in the formula so that it is significantly less drying to the hair than the solvents normally used."

While there are hair-coloring options that utilize more natural ingredients and contain less of the highly toxic chemicals traditionally associated with hair dye, they are certainly not without risk. These are difficult decisions for many women to make, and my hope is that in time, we'll see better options offered.

## Choosing Safer Personal Care Products

To help you make safer choices, the Environmental Working Group has created an extensive database of products they have tested for safety. Their **Skin Deep** database rates over 80,000 products for safety. You can search for products by name, or by category, such as sunscreen, makeup, skin care, hair care, nail care, fragrances, oral care, and products for men, babies, and moms. They also have a mobile app to help you at the store!

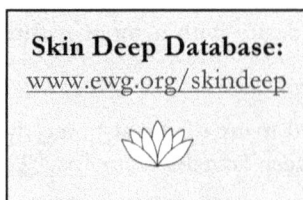

---

**Skin Deep Database:**
www.ewg.org/skindeep

---

We all have our favorite personal care products. If you are curious about how safe they are, visit the EWG's Skin Deep database or do some of your own research. If you're not comfortable with what you find, you may want to try some safer options. Fortunately we have many wonderful options to choose from today. Be kind to yourself and your family. ❤

## True Beauty

*"For attractive lips, speak words of kindness.*
*For lovely eyes, seek out the good in people.*
*For a slim figure, share your food with the hungry.*
*For beautiful hair, let a child run his or her fingers through it once a day.*
*For poise, walk with the knowledge that you never walk alone.*
*The beauty of a woman is not in the clothes she wears, the figure that she carries or the way she combs her hair.*
*The beauty of a woman must be seen from in her eyes, because that is the doorway to her heart, the place where love resides."*
*Audrey Hepburn*

Here are some **SHOPPING TIPS** for some popular personal care products (adapted from Environmental Working Group at www.ewg.org).

| Soap | **Avoid:** triclosan and triclocarban |
|---|---|
| Moisturizer & Lip Products | **Avoid:** Retinyl palmitate, retinyl acetate, retinoic acid and retinol in daytime products |
| Hand Sanitizers | **Pick:** ethanol or ethyl alcohol in at least 60% alcohol |
| Sunscreen | **Just say no:**<br>• SPF above 50<br>• Retinyl palmitate<br>• Aerosol spray and powder sunscreen<br>• Oxybenzone<br>• Added insect repellent<br>**Say yes to:**<br>• Hats and shade in mid-day sun<br>• Zinc Oxide or Titanium Dioxide as active ingredients, otherwise Avobenzone (at 3%)<br>• SPF 15 to 50, depending on your own skin<br>• Coloration, time outside, shade and cloud cover<br>• Use a lot and reapply frequently |
| Hair Care | **Avoid or limit:**<br>• Dark permanent hair dyes<br>• Chemical hair straighteners (especially keratin) |
| Toothpaste | **Avoid:** triclosan |
| Nails | **Avoid:**<br>• Formaldehyde or formalin in polish, hardeners or other nail products<br>• Toluene and Dibutyl phthalate (DBP) in polish<br>• Pregnant? Skip polish<br>**Choose:** Safer options at www.ewg.org/skindeep |
| Perfume, Cologne & Body Spray | **Avoid:**<br>• Diethyl phthalate<br>• "Fragrance" (listed as an ingredient) |
| Make-up | **Avoid:**<br>• Loose powders<br>• Vitamin A (listed as: retinol, retinyl palmitate, retinyl acetate) in skin and lip products<br>**Choose:**<br>Safer make-up - see "Skin Deep" database |

# 8 OTHER SOURCES OF TOXINS

## Non-Stick Cookware

We love non-stick pans, and it's no wonder since they're easy to cook with and the clean up is a breeze. Despite the advantages, these pans have been under fire for years because of the chemicals they can emit when cooking on higher heat. The non-stick repellent coating contains PFOA (perfluorooctanoic acid), a synthetic chemical that creates their slippery no-stick finish. These chemicals have been linked to cancer, liver damage and developmental problems. A study published in the *Journal of Clinical Endocrinology and Metabolism* in 2011 found that PFOA may cause early menopause.

These chemicals were found in the umbilical cord of newborns in the EWG studies we've previously talked about. The Johns Hopkins Bloomberg School of Public Health actually found PFOA in 100% of the newborns they examined in 2007. This is a clear example of how our lifestyle choices can impact future generations. While non-stick cookware is not the only source for PFOA exposure, it is a common one.

## Cast Iron Pans

If you've never owned a cast iron pan, then you're in for a real treat. A few years ago, I bought two cast iron skillets, a large family-sized one and a small one for 1-2 servings. I absolutely love these pans and use them so often that I leave them on my stove most of the time, primarily because they're so heavy to keep putting away.

There are many benefits to cooking in cast iron. From a culinary perspective, they conduct heat beautifully and they can go from stove to oven easily, making one-dish meals easy. They are fantastic for searing meat and chicken, as well as creating crispy potatoes and caramelized veggies. The real plus is that they are chemical-free and a great alternative to nonstick pans. While they don't leach chemicals, they may add a little iron to your food.

A well-seasoned cast iron pan requires less oil when cooking. "Seasoning" a new cast iron skillet is important to create a nonstick finish and prevent rust.

To season a new cast iron skillet:
- Start by washing your new pan with hot, soapy water, rinse well, and dry completely.
- Next, take a paper towel and rub some vegetable oil all over the entire pan, including the exterior.
- Place it upside down in a 350-degree oven and bake it for 1 hour. Place a sheet of foil underneath to catch any drips. Let it cool down in the oven completely.

Once seasoned, you should never use soap to clean your pan. All you'll need is a good stiff brush and some hot water. An alternative way to clean it is by rubbing it with salt, then rinse. Always be sure to dry your pan completely. You can season your pan whenever it appears to need it. With proper care, these pans will last a lifetime and they are practically indestructible.

## Other Healthy Options

Because cast iron is heavy, some people may prefer **carbon steel cookware,** which can weigh from one half to two thirds that of cast iron. It also seasons well and is cared for in the same way as cast iron, although soap is acceptable now and then as long as you thoroughly dry it.

While both cast iron and carbon steel are considered by most experts to be healthy types of cookware, they are not recommended when cooking acidic foods because they can give food a metallic taste. In these cases, you may want to consider an alternative such as **enameled cast iron** cookware, a high-quality **stainless steel,** or **ceramic** cookware.

While enameled cast iron is healthy cookware, it does tend to be very expensive. If you can afford a couple of pieces, you'll probably find that it's a great investment.

Many people feel that stainless steel is also a healthier choice for cooking. A good quality 18/10 stainless steel has a core of aluminum or copper (or both). While there is much controversy about cooking directly with either aluminum or copper, the stainless steel provides protection from direct contact with these metals while allowing for the excellent heat conductivity that they provide. Stainless steel cookware is best suited for liquids such as making sauces and soups since it does not have a non-stick surface.

Your choice of cookware is an important investment when you consider the impact that it has on your family's health. Buying a few good quality pieces when you can afford it will serve your family well for years to come.

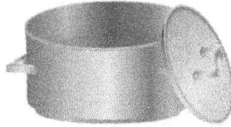

## Plastics

Plastics are everywhere. They hold our drinking water, line our canned goods, and even seal our healthiest foods. Some are eco-friendly and even appear to be safe for our kids. Others emit dangerous toxins during manufacturing, and some are suspected of causing harm, particularly to our children.

There are plenty of things you can do to reduce your exposure to plastic, like replacing your plastic water bottles with stainless steel ones, or using glass storage containers instead of plastic ones. Even so, you'll probably still be using a lot of plastic, so why not learn which ones are the most important ones to avoid, whenever possible.

## Know Your Plastics: Check the Resin Identification Code

If you want to control the amount of plastic you expose your family to, then I recommend you learn more about how to identify them so that you can make more informed decisions about the risks they pose. Plastics have a classification system that is printed on the bottom of most plastic bottles and food containers. This was developed in 1988 to help consumers and recyclers to properly recycle and dispose of the different types of plastics.

> **Safer Choices: 1, 2, 4 & 5**
> **Try to Avoid: 3, 6, & 7**

## Plastic #1: Polyethylene Terephthalate (PET)

Uses: Most commonly seen in thin, clear plastic water bottles, cooking oil, soft drinks, medicine jars, peanut butter jars, combs, beanbags, and rope.

Recycled PET: textiles, tote bags, carpet, fiberfill in winter clothing, plastic lumber, parking lot bumpers.

Safety: Considered safe, although they can leach toxic metal antimony during manufacturing. These plastic containers should never be reused, refilled or heated.

Canadian Study - 63 brands of bottled water produced in Europe and Canada found antimony concentrations >100x typical level of clean groundwater. (21) Bromine compounds found to leach into PET bottles have potential affect on central nervous system. (22)

## Plastic #2: High Density Polyethylene (HDPE)

Uses: This is the thicker, opaque or milkier plastic used for milk jugs, water jugs, juice bottles, motor oil, shampoos and conditioners, soap bottles, detergents, bleaches, and toys.

It is NEVER safe to reuse an HDPE bottle as a food or drink container if it didn't originally contain food or drink. However, they are safe to refill and reuse when they originally contained food/drink.

Recycled HDPE: fencing, plastic lumber, plastic crates (products similar to #1).

Safety: Considered a low-hazard but has been found to release estrogenic chemicals.

Study: 95% of all plastic products tested were positive for estrogenic activity, meaning they can potentially disrupt your hormones and even alter the structure of human cells, posing risks to infants and children. In this particular study, even products that claimed to be free of the common plastic toxicant bisphenol-A (BPA) still tested positive for other estrogenic chemicals.

## Plastic #3: Polyvinyl Chloride (PVC) - AVOID #3!

Uses: Most commonly found in cling wrap, bibs, mattress covers, squeeze bottles, some peanut butter jars, plumbing pipes, bags for bedding, deli and meat wrap, plastic toys, table cloths, and blister packs used to store medications. Plastic can be flexible or rigid.

Not often recycled.

Safety: Harmful if ingested.
PVC manufacturing releases dioxin into the environment, a dangerous carcinogen that accumulates in animals and humans. May also contain phthalates, including DEHP, a type of phthalate used as a plastics softener. Some phthalates are hormone disrupters that have been linked to possible birth defects and reproductive problems, including smaller penis size in boys and "gender-bending" chemicals that cause males of many species to become more female.

These chemicals have disrupted the endocrine systems of wildlife, causing testicular cancer, genital deformations, low sperm counts and infertility in a number of species, including polar bears, deer, whales, and otters.

PVC plant workers have higher cancer rates. Discard at recycling plant.

## Plastic #4: Low Density Polyethylene (LDPE)

Uses: LDPE is found in soft plastics that are flexible including bags for bread, newspapers, fresh produce, household garbage and frozen foods in addition to hot and cold cups and paper milk cartons.

These should be recycled, not thrown away.
Can use reusable shopping bags to replace some of these.

Safety: Considered low hazard. While LDPE does not contain BPA, it may pose risks of leaching estrogenic chemicals, similar to HDPE.

# Plastic #5: Polypropylene (PP)

Uses: Used to make hard, but flexible plastics, such as containers for yogurt, deli foods, ice cream, drinking straws, syrup bottles, salad bar containers, diapers, medications and takeout meal containers.
Recycle; don't throw away.

Safety: Considered one of the safer plastics. Has high heat tolerance so unlikely to leach chemicals, at least one study found that PP plastic ware used for laboratory studies did leach at least two chemicals (Science. 2008 Nov 7;322(5903):917).

# Plastic #6: Polystyrene (PS) - AVOID #6!

Uses: Polystyrene is found in rigid plastics such as opaque plastic forks and spoons. Includes Styrofoam, and used to make cups, plates, bowls, take-out containers, meat trays and more.

Safety: Polystyrene is known to leach styrene, a neurotoxin that can damage your nervous system and is linked to cancer.

Hot temperatures leach more styrene leaches from polystyrene containers, so using these for hot foods and beverages (such as hot coffee in a polystyrene cup) may be very dangerous.

# Plastic #7: Other (Includes Polycarbonate, Nylon, & Acrylic)

This is a catch-all symbol that includes polycarbonate, an important source of BPA, a known endocrine disrupter that has been found in most baby bottles, the lining of food and formula cans, and clear plastic cutlery.

This designation is used to describe products made from other plastic resins not described above, or made from a combination of plastics.

Code #7 includes newer, compostable green plastics made from rice, potatoes, corn, and tapioca, which should probably have their own code since they are safer bio-based plastics.

It's difficult to know the types of toxins that may be in #7 plastics, but they may contain BPA or the newer class of bisphenol known as bisphenol-S (BPS). Both BPA and BPS are endocrine disrupters and can interfere with or mimic the hormones in our bodies. In utero exposure to these compounds can lead to chromosomal errors, cause spontaneous miscarriage and DNA damage.

## BPA linked to Behavioral Problems

Everyone seems to know that BPA is something to be avoided due to toxicity. It is a polycarbonate that is classified as a #7 plastic.

According to a study led by researchers at Harvard School of Public Health, Cincinnati Children's Hospital and Medical Center, and Simon Fraser University in Vancouver, British Columbia published in 2011, exposure to bisphenol-A (BPA) in the womb is associated with more behavior and emotional problems at age 3, especially in young girls.

The study substantiates the findings of two prior studies also showing that exposure to BPA during pregnancy impacts child behavior. It is the first study to show that the impact of BPA exposure in utero is more significant than exposures that occur in childhood. Lead author of the study, Joseph Braun said, "Gestational, but not childhood BPA exposures, may impact neurobehavioral function, and girls appear to be more sensitive to BPA than boys."

Researchers advised clinicians to advise patients to reduce BPA exposure by avoiding canned and packaged food, thermal paper sales receipts, in addition to #7 recycling symbol polycarbonate bottles.

BPA is chemically similar to the hormone estrogen and is thought to mimic the same hormonal effects in the body, classifying it as part of a group of chemicals known as "endocrine disruptors."

Higher levels of BPA in urine have also been associated with an increased risk of obesity in children.

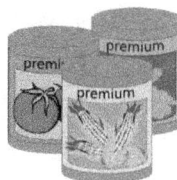

71

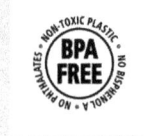
BPA-Lined Cans

BPA-lined cans have sparked a lot of attention in recent years, especially canned tomatoes because their acidic nature can significantly increase the likelihood of BPA leaching from the can.

A number of companies have stepped up and have chosen to phase out BPA liners with a goal of providing safer alternatives, despite their claim that the cost is higher. While we know there are serious risks associated with BPA, we don't always know about the safety of the new liners being used to replace them. As a pioneer in moving away from BPA linings, Eden Foods has posted some discussion on the their website about the safety of alternatives and their goals.

Because highly acidic foods, such as tomatoes pose a more challenging problem, some companies like Eden Foods are offering tomato products in jars. The lids of the jars can also contain BPA, although the amounts would likely be less. One company, Pomi, provides an alternative to cans by offering BPA-free boxed tomatoes.

Here are a few companies that have removed BPA from some or all of their can liners:

## Amy's

The company's website states: "We are pleased to announce that as of March 1, 2012, Amy's has completely transitioned to cans using no BPA in the formulation of its liner. Even though BPA is omnipresent in the environment from a multitude of sources, testing levels on our canned products with the new liner are showing reduced BPA levels of less than 1 part per billion."

## Muir Glen

Here is the response I received from the Company regarding the use of BPA:

"Muir Glen canned tomato products do not utilize BPA in product packaging. We know that some of our consumers have chosen to avoid BPA, so we had been looking for alternatives. Working with our can suppliers and can manufacturers, Muir Glen was able to develop and test a safe and viable alternative that does not use BPA for our canned tomato products. We began transitioning to those linings with the fall 2010 tomato pack – and we completed that transition with the 2011 tomato pack.

The new liners are a vinyl-based material. The safety of this can lining has been thoroughly tested. In addition to complying with requirements set forth by the FDA, Small Planet Foods board certified toxicologist has concurred with this assessment."

## Eden Foods

The Company's website states: "Since April of 1999, EDEN beans have featured a custom-made can lined with an oleoresinous c-enamel that does not contain the endocrine disrupter BPA. Oleoresin is a mixture of oil and resin extracted from plants such as pine or balsam fir.

Although we successfully achieved a BPA-free alternative for low-acid food such as beans, the canning industry has no suitable (in our opinion) can for high-acid food like tomatoes. After years of trying to realize one, Eden chose to move its canned tomatoes into amber glass jars to avoid BPA.

In 2011 Eden moved a third of its tomatoes to amber glass, away from cans. The cans still have a baked on r-enamel. Due to the acids in tomato, the lining is epoxy based and does contain a minute amount of BPA. It is however, in the 'non-detectable' range according to Eden's independent laboratory extraction tests. The test was based on a detection level of 5 ppb (parts per billion). Our goal is zero."

## Native Forest

The following products have BPA-free linings*:

Organic Coconut Milk (Classic and Light)
Organic Coconut Water
Organic Pineapple (all varieties)
Organic Tropical Fruits (Mango, Papaya Chunks & Tropical Fruit Salad)
Organic Mandarin Oranges
Organic Peaches
Organic Asian Pears
Organic Mangosteen
Organic Rambutan
Organic Grapefruit Segments
Organic Baby Corn
Organic Okra

*per email received September, 2014 from Edward & Sons, parent company.

## Trader Joe's

The Company sent the following response regarding the use of BPA:

"Below is a summary of TJ'S products and their BPA status:
Good: All our canned fish, canned chicken and canned beef are now in BPA-free cans EXCEPT: Sardines, Crab, Cherrystone Clams & Oysters.

Good: All our canned fruits and vegetables (including the All Canned Tomatoes and Organic Canned Pumpkin when it returns this Fall) are in BPA-free cans EXCEPT: Mandarins, Hatch Chilies, Artichokes, Organic Baked Beans.

Bad: All of our canned Soups and Stews (including Joe's Os) are in cans that DO have BPA.

Good: Coconut Milk, Organic Chili, Organic Soups all BPA FREE cans.

All of our suppliers of our BPA-lined canned products are working for a solution. We are handling this issue in the same manner as previous matters of concern: we're listening to the feedback our customers are providing and exploring options to put that feedback into place in a meaningful way."

## Westbrae

As of mid-2013, has labeled many of its cans as having non-BPA lining.

## Whole Foods

According to Whole Food's website:

"Whole Foods Market does not use register tapes in any US stores that are made with bisphenol-A (BPA). We work with our suppliers to strongly encourage the transition to non-BPA materials where functional alternatives exist. We actively pressure our canned good suppliers to transition to functional and safe alternative materials, and we are pleased that a number of national brands have begun the transition to non-BPA cans for a number of items. We have also been pursuing the use of alternatives to cans, such as glass jars and aseptic packaging (the paperboard cartons often used for broths or soy milks). It appears that many current alternatives will work well to protect low-acid foods but not higher-acid foods, so it's difficult to identify a single alternative that will work for all products. We also want to avoid using a material that is made without BPA but contains other estrogenic materials or toxins.

To date, we have done more than any other U.S. retailer to inform our customers and take action on the issue. We continue to closely examine the packaging materials used in our stores, and we will continue to search for the safest and most functional packaging materials for our stores."

## Other Retailers

Recently, both Wal-Mart and Toys R Us (also Babies R Us) have taken the lead by setting new guidelines to reduce phthalates in their toys. They plan to require independent third-party lab testing of batches of toys that are imported for sale in the U.S.

Other companies have announced that they plan to move away from the use of BPA in their packaging including Campbell Foods, Heinz, Hain Celestial Group and ConAgra.

# Tips for Reducing Plastic Exposure:

- If you microwave food or drink, try to **use glass or ceramic containers** instead of plastic & cover with **wax paper** instead of plastic wrap.
- Use **reusable shopping bags** for groceries.
- Buy food in **bulk** to avoid packaging.
- Bring your own mug for coffee when Styrofoam cups are used.
- Take your own non-plastic container to a restaurant for leftovers (especially **avoid Styrofoam** take-out containers which emit more styrene when food is hot).
- **Freeze foods in glass** as opposed to plastic bags.
- Replace your plastic kitchen storage containers with **glass or ceramic** containers.
- Filter your own water and use your own **water bottle** (preferably glass or heavy stainless steel).
- Avoid disposable utensils (especially with hot foods).
- Request no plastic wrap on your dry cleaning.
- **Avoid canned goods lined with BPA**. Some products are now being offered in boxes that pose less risk.
- Buy more fresh **local** foods from farmer's markets (less packaging and more nutritious).
- Wash your hands after handling **thermal-printed receipts**.
- If at all possible, try to purchase products that are not packaged in plastic or made from plastic.
- Remember to **check the bottom of plastic containers** and get to know the ones that are the most toxic.

**Try to avoid #3, #6 and most plastics labeled with #7.**

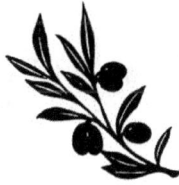

# 9 MAKING A DIFFERENCE

There's never been a time in history when so many kids are dealing with cancer, autism, allergies, asthma, and more. We cannot ignore the fact that our children are exposed to thousands of toxic chemicals as they go through the course of their every day lives. We each have countless opportunities to make a difference by being proactive and having a preventive mindset.

Because moms are the predominant decision makers when it comes to deciding which products and environments are safe and healthy for our children, we have tremendous market influence. By uniting together to spread awareness, voice our concerns to manufacturers, grocery stores, and policy makers, we can help to transform the marketplace to encourage safer products and environments for all children and for future generations.

While no one can do everything, everyone can do something to make a difference. May we all do our best to provide our children with a clean start in life. ❤

> *"The best and most beautiful things in this world cannot be seen or even heard, but must be felt with the heart." – Helen Keller*

# 10 RESOURCES & REFERENCES

Helpful Websites:

The Environmental Working Group: http://www.EWG.org
Provides breakthrough research to help consumers to make more informed decisions to live healthier lives in a healthier environment.

Grow Baby: www.growbabyhealth.com
Powerful nutritional management during preconception & pregnancy

Healthy Child, Healthy World: www.healthychild.org
To empower parents to take action and protect children from harmful chemicals.

US Health & Human Services: Household Products: www.householdproducts.nlm.nih.gov
Health & Safety information on household products

Consumer Product Safety Commission: www.cpsc.gov/en/Safety-Education/Safety-Guides/Home/
Home Safety Guide

Women's Voices For the Earth: www.womensvoices.org/wp-content/uploads/2011/11/Dirty-Secrets.pdf
Dirty Secrets: What's Hiding in Your Cleaning Products?

Consumer Product Safety Commission: www.cpsc.gov

Shaklee U.S.: shaklee.com
(Nancy's personal website: www.spiccia.myshaklee.com)
Products in Harmony with Nature

# References:

(1) Chemical analyses of 10 umbilical cord blood samples were conducted by AXY Analytical Services (Sydney, BC) and Flett Research Ltd. (Winnipeg, MB)

(2) M Lenoir, et al. Intense Sweetness Surpasses Cocaine Reward. PLoS ONE. 2007; 2(8): e698

(3) Journal of Environmental Monitoring (JEM) as reported by Rodale News (http://www.rodalenews.com/mercury-pollution-and-exposure?page=0,0)

(4) Freedman DS, Zuguo M, Srinivasan SR, Berenson GS, Dietz WH. Cardiovascular risk factors and excess adiposity among overweight children and adolescents: the Bogalusa Heart Study. *Journal of Pediatrics* 2007;150(1):12–17.

(5) Li C, Ford ES, Zhao G, Mokdad AH. Prevalence of pre-diabetes and its association with clustering of cardiometabolic risk factors and hyperinsulinemia among US adolescents: NHANES 2005–2006. *Diabetes Care* 2009;32:342–347.

(6) CDC. National diabetes fact sheet: national estimates and general information on diabetes and pre-diabetes in the United States, 2011[pdf 2.7M]. Atlanta, GA: U.S. Department of Health and Human Services.

(7) Daniels SR, Arnett DK, Eckel RH, et al. Overweight in children and adolescents: pathophysiology, consequences, prevention, and treatment. *Circulation* 2005;111;1999–2002.

(8) Office of the Surgeon General. The Surgeon General's Vision for a Healthy and Fit Nation. [pdf 840K], Rockville, MD, U.S. Department of Health and Human Services; 2010.

(9) Dietz WH. Overweight in childhood and adolescence. *New England Journal of Medicine* 2004;350:855-857.

(10) Freedman DS, Kettel L, Serdula MK, Dietz WH, Srinivasan SR, Berenson GS. The relation of childhood BMI to adult adiposity: the Bogalusa Heart Study. *Pediatrics*2005;115:22–27.

(11) Kushi LH, Byers T, Doyle C, Bandera EV, McCullough M, Gansler T, et al. American Cancer Society guidelines on nutrition and physical activity for cancer prevention: reducing the risk of cancer with healthy food choices and physical activity. *CA: A Cancer Journal for Clinicians* 2006;56:254–281.

(12) http://www.heart.org/HEARTORG/GettingHealthy/Make-the-Effort-to-Prevent-Heart-Disease-with-Lifes-Simple-7_UCM_443750_Article.jsp

(13) http://www.hsph.harvard.edu/nutritionsource/preventing-diabetes-full-story/

(14) American Association for Cancer Research (AARC) Cancer Progress Report 2014 http://cancerprogressreport.org/2014/Documents/AACR_CPR_2014.pdf

(15) The Canadian Journal of Veterinary Research, 2003

(16) "Report on Public Health Aspects of the Use of Bovine Somatotropin," issued March 15-16, 1999, and available from The European Commission—Food Safety.

(17) Holmes, Pollak, et. al. "Dietary Correlates of Plasma Insulin-like Growth Factor I and Insulin-like Growth Factor Binding Protein 3 Concentrations" Cancer Epidemiology, Biomarkers, and Prevention, Sept. 2002, p. 852-861; Chan, Stampfer, et. al."Plasma Insulin-like Growth Factor-I and Prostate Cancer Risk: A Prospective Study," Science, January, 1998, p 563-566; Yu, Jin, et. al, Insulin-like Growth Factors and Breast Cancer Risk in Chinese Women, Cancer

Epidemiology, Biomarkers, and Prevention, August 2002, p. 705-712.
(18) JAMA Pediatrics July 1, 2013
(19) Gray 1986, Schreurs 2004, Gomez 2005, Veldhoen 2006.
(20) Duty 2003, Hauser 2007, Swan 2005, Wolff 2008.
(21) Water Research, Volume 42, Issue 3, February 2008, Pages 551–556
(22) Environment International Volume 38, Issue 1, Jan 2012, Pgs 45–53
(23) www.ewg.org/bpa-in-store-receipts
(24) Source: EPA publication "Preventing Pests at Home": http://www.epa.gov/
(25) www.fda.gov/Food/FoodborneIllnessContaminants/Metals/ucm393070.htm
(26) Source: Healthychild.org
(27) Source: http://www.dailymail.co.uk/health/article-2232925/Pesticides-used-fruit-vegetables-putting-young-children-risk-cancer.html
(28) USDA Agricultural Marketing Service, 2010-2011 Pilot Study: Pesticide Residue Testing of Organic Produce, Nov. 2012
(29) Source: http://www.fda.gov/Food/FoodborneIllnessContaminants/Metals/ucm393070.htm
(30) Source: Dietaryguidelines.gov (Dietary Guidelines for Americans 2010, US Dept. of Agriculture and Dept. of Health and Human Services
(31) Source: www.fishwatch.gov/wild_seafood/outside_the_us.htm
(32) Organic Production Enhances Milk Nutritional Quality by Shifting Fatty Acid Composition: A United States–Wide, 18-Month Study Charles M. Benbrook, Gillian Butler, Maged A. Latif ,Carlo Leifert, Donald R. Davis Center for Sustaining Agriculture and Natural Resources, Washington State University, Pullman, Washington, United States of America, School of Agriculture, Food and Rural Development, Newcastle University, Northumberland NE, United Kingdom, Organic Valley/CROPP Cooperative/Organic Prairie, Lafarge, Wisconsin, United States of America
(33) Source: nepis.epa.gov (EPA 400-R-92-012 page 2, Targeting Indoor Air Pollution)
(34) Source: allergies.about.com; nsc.org; bt.cdc.gov
(35) 1890 Research & Extension Program at SC State University, August 2009
(36) Toronto Indoor Air Conference 1990
(37) FDA 2012 (CIR 2012) (fda.gov)
(38) FDA (Certech 2008) (fda.gov)
(39) FDA Certech 2008, IFRA 2010 (fda.gov)
(40) EPA: http://www.epa.gov/mercury/exposure.htm